Role Play and Clinical Communication

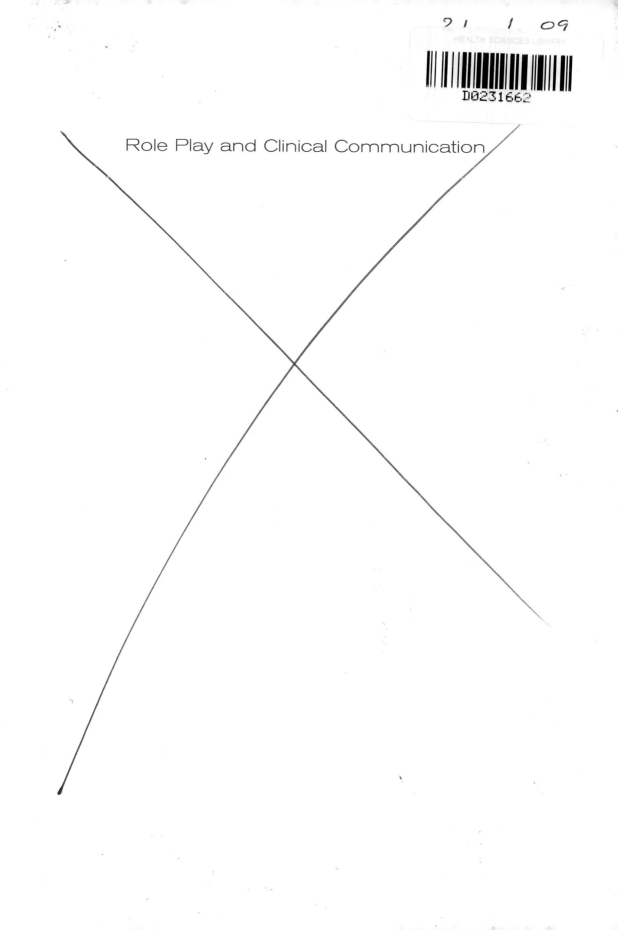

Role Play and Clinical Communication

LEARNING THE GAME

JOHN SKELTON

Director, Interactive Studies Unit
Department of Primary Care and General Practice
University of Birmingham

Radcliffe Publishing
Oxford • New York

Radcliffe Publishing Ltd
18 Marcham Road
Abingdon
Oxon OX14 1AA
United Kingdom

www.radcliffe-oxford.com
Electronic catalogue and worldwide online ordering facility.

British Library Cataloguing in Publication Data

A catalogue record for this book is available from the British Library.

ISBN-13: 978 1 84619 126 8

Typeset by Pindar New Zealand (Egan Reid), Auckland, New Zealand
Printed and bound by TJI Digital, Padstow, Cornwall, UK

Contents

Preface

This, the second of two books which look at aspects of the teaching of communication in a clinical setting, builds in particular on the work of the Interactive Studies Unit (ISU), based at the University of Birmingham Medical School, since the inception of the Unit in the early 1990s. The ISU has been involved in the teaching of many thousands of health professionals and students of the health professions, and certainly for me personally it has been a rewarding experience. Well, actually, no – that's not the point. The best of the students we've encountered over the years have frankly had the capacity to reaffirm our faith in human nature.

I owe debts to too many colleagues to name – the present core team within the Unit, the support of Departmental colleagues over the years, and that of colleagues within the West Midlands Postgraduate Workforce Deanery. However, I must single out Dr Kate Thomas, and the other founder members of the ISU, namely Professor Dave Fitzmaurice, Dr Phil Hammond and Dr Connie Wiskin, who has kindly agreed to co-author two chapters of this book, and whose energies, quick practical intelligence and huge enthusiasm are a marvel. Phil Hammond has moved on, but versions of many of the scenarios discussed here were created by him, and we all owe a considerable debt to his excellent eye for what would have clinical and educational value.

John Skelton
January 2008

About the authors

John Skelton is Director of the Interactive Studies Unit (ISU) at the University of Birmingham Medical School, where he is Professor of Clinical Communication. He is also Associate Dean for Educational Quality, and Director of the Medical School Education Unit. John is a literature graduate who, before getting involved in medical education, worked as a language teacher, teacher educator and applied linguist in Spain, Oman, Singapore and the UK. He still maintains his interest in education overseas, and has undertaken short consultancies in two dozen countries.

Connie Wiskin is Deputy Director of the Interactive Studies Unit (ISU) and Senior Lecturer in Clinical Communication. Connie set up the role play team at the University of Birmingham Medical School in 1991, and has remained committed to medical education since then. She has a background in humanities, and her research field is interactive summative assessment. Connie has presented her work on teaching and assessment methodologies internationally, and has produced a number of nationally available video/DVD training packages.

I mentioned my debt to my family in the Preface to the first of this two-book series, and it remains constant. *JS*

With thanks to my dad, Danny Wiskin, for getting me started. *CW*

What's the sign of someone's understanding a game? Must he be able to recite the rules? Isn't it also a criterion that he can play the game, i.e. that he does in fact play it, even if he's baffled when asked for the rules? Is it only by being told the rules that the game is learnt and not also simply by watching it being played? Of course a man will often say to himself while watching 'oh, so that's the rule'; and he might perhaps write down the rules as he observes them; but there's certainly such a thing as learning the game without explicit rules.

(Wittgenstein L. On the game of language. In: Rhees R, editor. *Philosophical Grammar*. Oxford: Oxford University Press; 1974. p. 62)

CHAPTER 1

Introduction

Instruction, Madam, is the pill; amusement is the gilding.

(Samuel Richardson, *Letters*[1])

The game of education

This is a book about certain aspects of simulation in clinical education. At its heart is a discussion of the use of role play in the teaching of communication and other issues, and I would like at the outset to be careful about how much – or how little – I am claiming originality for what I say. The kind of work I describe in this book is routine in clinical (particularly medical) education, it is often done exceptionally well, and the nuts and bolts of putting it into effect have been well described.[2] However, what doesn't happen particularly well or often is an attempt to put this kind of activity into its broader educational context, or to tease out its roots in the traditions of language in education. I shall discuss the latter point at some length, because without an understanding of the kind of language associated with the classroom, it is easy to miss the similarity between the professional language one tries to develop in students of the health professions, and the kind of language that is used by teachers – and it is easy therefore to miss the way that role-play exercises mirror the language of the lesson during which they take place. The doctor, the teacher and the role player do certain things in rather similar ways, and so too does the successful student.

I should also say that the book is not at all concerned with the use of clinical skills laboratories and the sophisticated equipment found in them which, from the days of Resusci Anne onwards, have enabled students to become more confident and dextrous (Cooper and Taqueti[3] offer a brief historical review of developments in such areas). Rather, I attempt to use role play as an entry-point for a more broad-based consideration of clinical education as a construct, as in some sense a product of artifice. The companion to this book (*Language and Clinical Communication: this bright Babylon*) was an extended exploration of the Chomskyean metaphor of 'surface' and 'depth' in language,[4] and by extension, education. This book is concerned similarly with what has been called – although the phrase is much less famous than Chomsky's – 'the language game of teaching'[5] and the game of role play and simulation in a clinical setting.

Bellack and colleagues picked up the 'game' analogy from Wittgenstein. The idea appears in *The Blue and Brown Books*[6] (transcripts of notes taken from Wittgenstein's lectures dating from the 1930s), and is pursued in *Philosophical Investigations*.[7] Above all, Wittgenstein is concerned with the relationship between words and their meanings. It is not enough to know a word, Wittgenstein argues in *Philosophical Investigations* – one must also know what the word is for:

> When one shows someone the king in chess and says: 'This is the king', this does not tell him the use of this piece – unless he already knows the rules of the game up to this last point . . .

For Wittgenstein, the fundamental problem with philosophy was its focus, as Hacker puts it,[8] 'on forms of expression rather than their use in the stream of life.' As any contemporary linguist would phrase it after Hymes,[9] it is wrong to focus on language *usage* (in the abstract) at the expense of language *use* (in fact) – or, as Wittgenstein states in *Philosophical Investigations*, 'The meaning of a word is its use in the language.'

Thus, in the abstract, without context, a sentence like 'The grass is long' is a statement about, well, the length of the grass. Provide it with a context, and it might mean 'Didn't you say you would definitely cut it this weekend?' or 'How can you play golf on a surface like this?' or any number of other things. Or, although we understand the difference between a compulsion and a choice, between what you *must* do and what you *want* to do, we are nevertheless too polite to say to our hosts, at the end of the evening, 'I want to leave.' We say we *must* leave, we affect surprise at the lateness of the hour, we talk of babysitters, the long road home, how early we are obliged to get up. But we know the rules – we cannot say we're leaving because we never wanted to come in the first place, we've put in the bare minimum length of stay, and now we've had enough.

So, then, we must understand the rules of chess in order to know what the meaning of 'the king' is. 'A king', we might say, 'is a piece which moves in such and such a way.' But this tells us little. Beyond this decontextualised piece of knowledge, and in order for us to begin to understand why this matters, we must add more information. That the object of chess is to checkmate the king – that the freedom of movement of the king is so restricted that a lot of game strategy is based on the defensive measures necessary to secure one's own king . . . and so on. Our understanding of the term 'king' as it is used in chess, we might say, grows as our understanding of the game of chess itself grows. In exactly the same way, a cardiologist's understanding of a phrase like 'His cholesterol is high' develops throughout their career.

All uses of language, from this analogy, may be considered as games, in the sense that there are certain conventions in all aspects of language use, in all settings, which must be followed, and many, many more which are typically followed. And, as Bellack and his colleagues pointed out, the classroom is also a setting, and has its rules. (I should stress here that the purpose of Bellack and his colleagues was to take Wittgenstein's metaphor to its limits, and to describe what they observed in the classroom – '*not* (their emphasis) *as a prescriptive guide to teacher behaviour.*')

Or at any rate, each setting has its tendencies – the word 'rule' perhaps gives the wrong impression. This is where the analogy with a game like chess breaks down. In chess, if one 'breaks the rules' by attempting to move the king two squares rather than one, then the game cannot continue. The rule breaker is presumably disqualified, and the game is at an end. There are rules of ordinary language which absolutely must be adhered to in a classroom, or in most settings, for the game to continue (e.g. for the conversation to be sustained). For example, don't insult the person you are speaking to, and don't hit them. However, these rules are so obvious that they are normally beside the point. What is of much greater interest is to specify the things which are less obvious, although in doing so you begin to talk of what often happens, not of what must happen. It is part of the social function of language to provide us with language norms through which we can talk to each other without causing offence. And it is part of its creative function to allow these norms to be broken for any number of reasons. One may offer an apparent insult to a friend ('You're such an idiot!') as an indicator of intimacy, and so on. The person who is a poor judge of when and how these norms can be breached is perceived as odd, or eccentric, or unconventional. The person who is an excellent judge of these matters will gain a reputation for being inventive, creative, or even something of a poet.

The rules of the game of teaching are one set of conventions, which I shall explore in some detail. The rules of the game of consulting with patients present us with another set which, as I shall try to argue, closely resemble those of teaching. The rules of the game of clinical role play are poorly understood, but straddle these two worlds.

Life is full of professional occasions. If we are teachers we need to interact with students, and if we are health professionals we need to interact with patients. But whoever we are, we also interact with the waiter who asks us whether we want to order wine, the garage mechanic who tells us we need new tyres, and so on, and such interactions are no less the result of language conventions. They are games in the restricted sense that they are played according to rules (or to tendencies), but they are life itself in all of its quotidian humdrum guise, and in that sense the game is as real as it gets. Yet in such exchanges we adopt social roles (as we inevitably call them), we do a kind of formal linguistic dance round each other, signalling status, level of formality, and the like. And – as I observe I have inadvertently done in this paragraph – we might end up talking of 'reality' as a 'guise.'

Simulation as an educational tool

Simulation – as employed in teaching – is something quite different, at one level. However, we should be aware that when we use role play to develop a medical student's communication skills, we are using simulation to teach him or her to play the role of 'doctor' more effectively.

This brings us to educational simulation itself. It is normal to trace educational simulations back to the development of board games which mirror war and the manoeuvres of war, so that – once more – the analogy is among other things with chess, although Wei Qi (better known in the west through its Japanese name, Go) probably pre-dates it. Cohen and Rhenman – who give an excellent historical overview[10] of simulation up to the early 1960s, on which I draw for the next couple of paragraphs – point out:

> As is well recognized by the students of the history of chess, this and other similar board games were at a very early stage used as symbolic equivalents to warfare. From this beginning it was probably a very short step to attempt to use these games for planning and training purposes.

Such games became more elaborate through Europe in the eighteenth century, culminating in Schleswig in the 1790s, with a game developed by George Venturini, played over 3600 painted squares. 'Unfortunately', as has dryly been pointed out, 'the complexity of the game grew to such an extent that it became almost impossible to play or referee it'[11] (translation by this author).

From here to the elaborate war games undertaken by modern armies is a short step, and from there to the use of simulation in other contexts is an equally short one. The American Management Association (AMA) was looking at this by the 1950s:[12]

> In the war games conducted by the Armed Forces, command officers of the Army, Navy and Air Force have an opportunity to practice decision-making creatively in a myriad of hypothetical yet true-to-life competitive situations. Moreover they are forced to make decisions in areas outside their own specialty; a naval communications officer for example may play the role of a task force commander.
>
> Why then shouldn't businessmen have the same opportunity? Why shouldn't a vice-president say in charge of advertising have a chance to play the role of company president for fun and for practice?

'For fun and for practice.' There has always been a strong link between the idea of context and simulation, and the idea of fun. Contexts, it is argued, provide meaning, and therefore contexts motivate. They provide both instruction and amusement.

Since the 1950s there has been a huge increase in the use of simulation in all disciplines, not least as a result of the developing sophistication of computer simulations, and of the understanding of how these might be used in teaching (see, for example, the journal *Simulation and Gaming*).

There are three central points to make at this stage. First, the history of simulation for educational and training purposes is a history of the development of complex contexts. Simulations are typically pared down to some degree, but they have always been detailed enough to create an illusion of reality. Indeed, if they lack this kind of depth, we deny them the name of simulation. This, for instance, is the original AMA game, as it was briefly described at the time:[12]

> The game consists of five teams of three to five persons each. These companies produce a single product which they sell in competition with each other in a common market . . . There are six types of decisions which each team must make every quarter [i.e. every simulated quarter of a year]. They must choose a selling price for their product, decide how much to spend for marketing activities, determine their research and development expenditures, select a rate of production, consider whether or not to change plant capacity and decide whether marketing research information about competitors' behavior should be purchased.

It is the rich context of simulations which drives them. Within the kind of simulation that is dealt with in this book — role-play activity for health professionals and students of the health professions – the richness of the context should be made as clear as possible to the participants.

Secondly, the clinician's instinct, faced with complex data, is Holmesian. That is to say, it is Sherlock Holmes' brilliance to look at the mysterious and unsorted data of the crime scene, and to identify possible hypotheses ('I have devised seven separate explanations, each of which would cover the facts as far as we know them', he says in *The Adventure of the Copper Beeches*[13]). These possibilities are closed down as evidence accumulates. So it is the doctor's task to identify, seize and work with the single truth which is in there somewhere. This is the essence of the account that Greenhalgh gives us in what has become a *locus classicus* of narrative-based medicine, 'Dr Jenkins's hunch':[14]

> I got a call from a mother who said her little girl had had diarrhoea and was behaving strangely. I knew the family well, and was sufficiently concerned to break off my Monday morning surgery and visit immediately.

This, Greenhalgh tells us, is 'a comment made by a general practitioner . . . which I have expanded into a hypothetical example.' The point is that the doctor picked up on the use of the unexpected word 'strangely' – rather than 'poorly', 'off-colour' or the like – and felt that there was something there which needed his immediate attention. And sure enough, the child had meningococcal meningitis.

It's a powerful story. However, we should be careful about the extent to which we claim that this is the way that narratives are, and certainly we should be careful about assuming that this is what they are designed to be. Dr Jenkins's hunch exemplifies precisely the type of approach one finds in detective literature – that is, literature as puzzle, and the hero (like the doctor) as problem solver. However, literary narratives ('literary' in the sense of being written as 'Literature' with a capital 'L') are not like this. They are concerned with offering visions of the world as it is – irreducibly complex but presented as the product of a coherent vision. Great literature is by its nature ambiguous. There may be an unequivocal motive for Professor Plum's attack with the lead piping in the library (it was love what made him do it, let's say). There is no certain answer to the question 'What was Iago's motive?'

To say that simulations are designed to be complex is to say that they are designed to be ambiguous, therefore, and not (or not usually) to have a single correct answer. Where medicine in particular is concerned, they will introduce students to a world in which problems are *managed* rather than *solved*. It is the nature of medicine that a single choice must be made (to treat or not, to treat in this way or that). However, it is the nature of simulation to insist on the ambivalence of the background against which these choices are made.

Thirdly, I tried to argue in *Language and Clinical Communication* that 'communication skills training', considered as a set of variably well-defined behaviours such as 'open questions', provided the student with a bedrock of skills which were appropriate to be aware of and to reflect on, but that the communication skills syllabus soon petered out. One reason for this is that there really isn't a great deal of meat on the bone, as far as most students are concerned. Not at least if the metaphorical meat we are looking for is thought to consist of rules for the game of communication. What is general enough to be a rule ('Don't hit your patient') is often too obvious to teach, and much of what is not too obvious to teach is insufficiently general to constitute a rule. The right thing to say depends too much on who does the saying, and who does the hearing, and under what circumstances. Beyond the obvious, that is, good communication differs in different contexts.

Thus, where relatively few context-free rules can be offered, the point of the simulation is to offer a three-dimensional setting in which choices about *what* to say and *how* can be informed by situation. Words have meaning as they are used.

The limits of a curriculum

The context in which most clinical communication skills training is undertaken is very restricted, at least as the phrase 'clinical communication skills' is normally used. Fundamentally, it refers to health professional and patient/client interaction, it concentrates on broadly emotional issues, and it advocates a model developed principally in primary care and other specialties – such as cancer care – where talking therapy may be of clear benefit. Also, typically, each simulated interaction is with a patient who is conjured from the air for a single meeting, and never seen again.

Yet everyone involved in the delivery of clinical education and training is aware of the fact that aspects of communication matter in many settings. One aspect of 'communication' which most doctors have to deal with, for instance, is teaching. It is an expectation of *Tomorrow's Doctors*,[15] the General Medical Council statement about what medical students should learn, that they have a basic understanding of the nature of teaching and learning:

> Graduates must understand the principles of education as they are applied to medicine. They will be familiar with a range of teaching and learning techniques and must recognise their obligation to teach colleagues. They must understand the importance of audit and appraisal in identifying learning needs for themselves and their colleagues.

Similarly, there is the issue of 'broadening the notion of competence' developed in the UK in the wake of the Bristol Royal Infirmary report[16]:

Clearly, healthcare professionals must be technically competent to do the task they profess to do, but technical competence is no longer sufficient, if indeed it ever was. A major lesson of our Inquiry is that there are a number of non-technical, non-clinical skills of doctors, nurses and managers which are crucially important to the care of patients. We have identified six key areas. They appear to have been relatively neglected in the education and training of healthcare professionals in the past. They must not be in the future. They are:

- skills in communicating with patients and with colleagues;
- education about the principles and organisation of the NHS;
- how care is managed, and the skills required for management;
- the development of teamwork;
- shared learning across professional boundaries;
- clinical audit and reflective practice; and
- leadership.

All of these issues – not just 'talking to patients and colleagues', but also leadership and the like – have a straightforward communication angle. And for that matter, the broader notion of clinical competence, or the list of competences that it subsumes, is as good a reminder as any of the way in which 'communication' as a curriculum issue can be embedded in a wide variety of settings.

What we have at this stage, then, is a view of communication as something which can usefully be practised within the setting of a simulation which is designed to be particularised. These settings will therefore present a very specific and detailed situation. And we also have a view of the communication curriculum as something which can permeate a wider set of non-clinical competences.

Both of these conditions imply an approach to the delivery of teaching which starts small (the single role play, the single competence), yet which has the capacity for indefinite expansion – and which also aims to give the learner the opportunity to reflect on the individual case, and to build generalisations from it.

And this, to a substantial extent, is the educational ethos of all kinds of case-based curriculum design. It therefore sits very comfortably within a problem-based learning (PBL) curriculum.

Things to do, people to see . . . What is a syllabus, anyway?

A few points about 'curricula' in general are relevant here.

There is wide variation in what people mean when they use the word 'curriculum.' Sometimes it means a bigger unit than a syllabus, and sometimes (I shall use it this way) it means much the same thing as a syllabus. However, there is another more important point. Strictly speaking, a curriculum should specify *what* ought to be taught. These days, this list of 'what to teach' will end in a series of statements about the attributes that learners will have as and when they successfully complete the curriculum (for example, 'Students will be able to percuss the chest'). And these statements will be as precise as they can be made, where possible by specifying them as a list of behaviours which can be evidenced ('Students will be able to get a blood pressure reading agreed as "accurate" as a result of an experienced clinician obtaining the same result within x minutes to an accuracy of y%', if one wants to be really elaborate).

In this sense, a curriculum ought to be easily distinguishable from the methodologies through which it is delivered. Just as a curriculum tells us *what* to teach, so a methodology tells us *how* to do this. The trouble is that curricula tend to be designed with certain methodologies already in mind. PBL is a simple example of this. Although the phrase 'PBL curriculum' is routinely used, 'problem-based learning' is, after all, actually a label for a set of methodologies, not for a set of things to learn. As a matter of fact, then, PBL is understood to mean both an organisation of content into 'problems', and delivery through self-study, access to tutors, and all the rest of it.

Moreover, teaching and learning are notoriously not the same. What the curriculum specifies as the material to be taught is not what the student will learn – not just because they will misunderstand and learn badly, or forget and learn partially, but because all students come to the curriculum with different previous experiences. Any new learning has to be sorted in the context of previous learning, which will give it a slightly different flavour from student to student. And the experience of learning will expose the learner to influences of which the curriculum writers in their wisdom are aware, but either do not or cannot articulate. This kind of thing is what we mean by talking of a hidden curriculum, and such external influences are presumed to be particularly at stake in the education of clinicians, where the presence of potential role models is much discussed.

So what is not hidden? What can be specified? Well, any curriculum represents an attempt to organise something or other. Education rests on the assumption that organised exposure of some sort works better than simple exposure to the setting where an activity takes place. You cannot effectively learn to be a doctor *just* by hanging around a hospital (although this is notoriously what a lot of medical students do on placements). The data that one obtains through mere exposure must be organised. As a single example, Lenin (reported on here by one of his more positive biographers[17]), realising that his book knowledge of English 'bore only a remote resemblance to the native product', set about learning the language:

> He went wherever he could hear English spoken, to pubs, to Hyde Park, to all
> sorts of meetings. Crowding up front, he listened carefully to every word, and
> watched the lip movements of speakers. In addition he hired two English teachers
> whom he taught Russian in exchange for English lessons.

Exposure and tuitions. Teaching is a question of identifying similarities, representing these as general principles, and bundling them up together.

The relationship between *exposure* to the learning setting – to the ward, or to the language used in pubs – and conscious learning of the rules of the games one sees played in such circumstances is at the heart of educational debate. At what one might call very loosely the more traditional extreme, it's all rules and no exposure. At the other extreme, there is an obvious danger that the curriculum will become no more than a specification of a set of things to do, a calendar of occasions on which exposure happens. Hence the teacher's natural instinct to make generalisations, to bundle exposure up into truths about the topic that is being taught.

The simplest things to bundle up are pieces of knowledge – a list of dates in history, the chemical properties of the inert gases, Newton's second law, and so on. A list of facts, therefore, might form the basis of the curriculum – the answer to the question 'What shall I teach my students?' However –Wittgenstein's game again – these things, the actual words in which Newton's second law is phrased, mean nothing without context, just as the rule about moving the king in chess means nothing without a sense of what implications this has for the conduct of the game.

This has always really been understood. Learning has never really been perceived as, say, the decontextualised rote learning of facts for their own sake. For example, the history of Latin teaching in the UK is often referred to as a means of exemplifying all that was wrong with such learning ('amo, amas, amat') of facts. However, the *reason* for the study of Latin was much wider. Dorothy Sayers, best known as the creator of the sleuth Lord Peter Wimsey, sums up some of the more educationally obvious aspects of this in a self-consciously provocative if not slightly eccentric essay from the 1940s, which was much reprinted for many years[18] (the essay was first given as a talk at Oxford University, and has since been printed more than once by the National Review, and elsewhere):

> I will say at once, quite firmly, that the best grounding for education is the Latin
> grammar. I say this, not because Latin is traditional and mediaeval, but simply
> because even a rudimentary knowledge of Latin cuts down the labor and pains
> of learning almost any other subject by at least fifty percent. It is the key to the

vocabulary and structure of all the Teutonic languages, as well as to the technical vocabulary of all the sciences and to the literature of the entire Mediterranean civilization, together with all its historical documents.

In a similar fashion, classical Chinese civil service entrance exams famously involved the study of poetry, but here too we may assume that the learning by heart of great poetry was not an end in itself, but evidence of an intellectually and emotionally sophisticated mind, such as would deal wisely with the problems of state.

However, education cuts deeper than this. Its power to influence is well understood. Here is a rather more sinister take on the merits of chanting by rote in class:[19]

> We must allow an effect to the continual impact of precept. Whether as the master's exhortation, as oft-quoted injunction, as memorized text, or as schoolroom motto, a persistent suggestion as to conduct, provided it really strike the attention and be brought home by illustration and instance, ought to count for something. The mere droning or dinning of maxims is perhaps vain, but that which is really *taught* certainly tends to *sink in* . . .
>
> Let us not forget that the immemorial advice of stationary societies to preserve their ancient order has been to make certain traditional wisdom the sole subject of study. The mere learning by rote of Analects, or Vedas, or Koran, or Thorah has been for thousands of years not unjustly deemed of great effect in molding character and fixing habits of thought.

These days, in the clinical professions, the custom is to divide education into knowledge, skills and attitudes. So, in contemporary jargon, we might argue that the knowledge-based curriculum (answering an exam question such as 'List the Ten Commandments') and the methodologies that accompany it ('mere learning by rote') have an effect on attitude. Such is 'the continual impact of precept.'

The difference in contemporary education, however, is that we no longer feel we can list only the facts and let the meanings – the links to other educational opportunities in Sayers' suggestion, and to moral control in Ross's – take care of themselves. We feel the need to make such things explicit, and it's in the explicit discussion of them that we find the meaning of the language games we play when we talk about being a health professional.

However, such things are a lot easier to discuss than to specify formally. Attempts to do so can simply look like attempts to shape the breeze as it passes.

Take 'experiential learning', for example. Rather than learn the multiplication tables by rote, we could do some practical mathematics. So we might send everyone to the race track and invite them to use their knowledge of multiplication to beat the bookies ('If I put £10 on a horse at 6–1 and it wins, and I put half the proceeds on another at 15–2 and it loses, how much do I have left?'). What would students learn under such circumstances? It's hard to say. Experiential learning, by its very nature, has unpredictable consequences. In this example, clearly there is the potential for learning about the surrounding moral issues, and psychological issues, and – as our students thumb a lift home in the rain – about the nature of probability and risk.

In other words, it is the nature of the PBL curriculum to draw attention to the existence of the hidden curriculum, and to specify it, inevitably, in a very imprecise way. The basic unit of currency in PBL is the problem, and it can sometimes be fairly difficult to atomise it further, at least with any confidence. This is a difficulty, but perhaps it is one we should live with. After all, the basic unit of medicine is, if not a 'problem' in the PBL sense, at least a single case. A clinician's life very often involves seeing a long series of single cases, each presenting problems – again in the non-technical sense – that are similar in general yet different in particulars, one after the other.

This is, in a sense, the real logic behind the PBL movement. It mirrors the professions, and if it comes to that, it is logistically easier to provide learning opportunities if course designers can think in terms of providing cases rather than abstract principles. A contrast is generally drawn between the traditional, top-down, deductive curriculum and the new, bottom-up, inductive curriculum. The former has Professor Boresbynight standing up and saying 'The principal characteristics of macular degeneration are . . .', with eager students subsequently observing as they move from patient to patient that this is all true. The latter has Dr Upandatem (much younger, I think) saying 'Observe Mr Patel, and Mrs Smith . . . what do they have in common? What pattern do you see?'

The latter way of looking at things is broadly mentalist (for a discussion of this, see *Language and Clinical Communication*) – from exposure to a series of similar situations in which we encounter similar data, we induce a general pattern. However, the point is that this is to an extent happenstance. The nature of healthcare is that it is case based anyway.

And this is also the context of role play. A role play is a case, clearly, except that it is simulated. For this reason, role play as an activity fits well with the healthcare professions because the unit of currency is familiar both to the practising clinician and to the PBL educator. A role play is not a 'problem' in the sense that PBL exponents use that term, although it can very usefully be made the base for a formal PBL exercise, but it does share the same three preconceptions. Context provides meaning. The healthcare professions are best viewed as case based. Students learn through the accumulation of particular examples.

Education is simulation

Education is not 'real' in one obvious sense. It takes place for the purpose of learning, not doing. However, attempts have been made – and have always been made – to offer a veneer of realism. And by this, often, what is meant is a veneer of context.

Thus the complex pill of arithmetical abstraction was introduced to generations of puzzled children wrapped in the gilding of surreal fictional narratives, a series of worlds in which Tom attempted to fill his bathtub at x gallons per minute while neglecting (Inattention? A caprice?) to insert the plug, an aberration which undermined his efforts at a rate of y pints per second. Or, as I recall, a world in which a footballer might advance across the face of the opposing goal and pause for a second to calculate the moment at which the gap between the goalkeeper and the near post was at its widest, and therefore most favourable for a shot. The goalkeeper (marked x in your textbook) was, perhaps, lost in higher mathematical abstractions of his own, and assumed to be static throughout. Similarly, foreign language students in the UK have routinely been sent out on the streets for years, perhaps bolstered by a questionnaire devised in class, to help them to 'find out' about some topic of debate or other by talking to 'real people.' I have been asked myself under these circumstances, as a stray individual walking along the street and approached by happenstance. As I too was a language teacher at the time, I was able to reflect on the solipsistic nature of the educational world.

Nevertheless, context has often been perceived as important. As is so often the case, the more articulate elements of the tradition as it has surfaced in recent eras can be traced back to John Dewey, who phrased the issue partly as a philosophical one – a matter of not distinguishing between mind and body and beyond that, therefore, between the world of the classroom and the world beyond. Here is one of Dewey's many statements about context (versus rote learning), linked here with an emphasis on the process of enquiry rather than the knowledge which the product might be. An apparent emphasis, that is, on 'learning for life', on 'learning by doing', and among other things in consequence on project-based learning:

> Moreover by following, in connection with problems selected from the material of ordinary acquaintance, the methods by which scientific men have reached

their perfected knowledge, [the learner] gains independent power to deal with material within his range, and avoids the mental confusion and intellectual distaste attendant upon studying matter whose meaning is only symbolic. Since the mass of pupils are never going to become scientific specialists, it is much more important that they should get some insight into what scientific method means than that they should copy at long range and second hand the results which scientific men have reached. Students will not go so far, perhaps, in the 'ground covered', but they will be sure and intelligent as far as they do go.[20]

Beyond Dewey also is the influence of William James and the pragmatists, for whom knowledge had value insofar as it was useful. And in general the weight of tradition and debate has been, for around 100 years, against abstract learning, and in favour of the provision of context. In more recent times, the thrust of educational ideas such as Gardner's Multiple Intelligences[21] can equally imply that the richness of the context provided is central to the learning experience. There is at one level an appeal to the cognitive advantages of contextualisation. At another level, there is an appeal to the psychological, to the motivational power – the 'fun', as we have seen – of context, authenticity, 'reality.'

In the end, however, the classroom is not real. Learning, as we saw, has a structure that the world does not have. Learning medicine does not happen merely through exposure – or at any rate, it would happen infinitesimally slowly as, step by step, the facts of medical knowledge were rediscovered. Learning is about grouping things together, and about short cuts – the short cuts provided by books, discussions with experts, and the generalisations of the classroom. And, at an entirely different level, the goalkeeper is fictitious, and – simulation being a difficult art – does not behave as a goalkeeper should. Even the man on the street turns out to be just another teacher, if it comes to that. And if the patient is real, and the heart murmur is real, the reason for the student listening to it is not the same as the reason why he or she needs to develop the ability to hear it – one is concerned with classroom practice, and the other with the practice of medicine.

From which I would invite you to conclude that simulation does not imply realism. The role of the simulator (role player, course designer) is not to be the same as the world. In a sense, that is what the world is for. Rather it is to offer opportunities to practise the relevant skills, to apply the relevant knowledge, and to reflect on the relevant attitudes, in as effective a manner as possible. The point about role players, if they are sufficiently skilled, is that they are not patients, but something else, a point which is only now beginning to be understood.[22]

There is a cautionary tale about illusion, course design and authenticity in education, which every educator should hear. When the playwright Eugene

Ionesco was a young man, living in Paris, he tried to learn English using the *Assimil* textbooks which were much in vogue at the time. As so often happens, the course designers' attention was focused on the formal teaching points to be delivered rather than the authenticity of either the language or the storyline. Ionesco was so struck by this, and the inconsequential dialogue it gave rise to, that he wrote what he called 'A pseudo-play', *The Bald Prima Donna*[23] – which was originally in fact to be called *L'Anglais Sans Peine*. Here is an extract, concerning the death of one Bobby Watson:

> *Mr Smith:* . . . He made the best looking corpse in Great Britain. And he never looked his age. Poor old Bobby! He'd been dead four years and he was still warm. A living corpse if ever there was one. And how cheerful he always was.
>
> *Mrs Smith:* Little Bobby, poor darling!
>
> *Mr Smith:* What do you mean, 'Poor darling'?
>
> *Mrs Smith:* I was thinking about his wife. Her name was Bobby, like his. As they had the same name, when you saw them together, you could never tell one from the other. It was really only after he died that you could tell which was which. But fancy, even now, there are still people who mix her up with her dead husband when they offer their condolences. Did you know her, dear?
>
> *Mr Smith:* I only saw her once, quite by chance, at Bobby's funeral.
>
> *Mrs Smith:* I've never seen her. Is she nice-looking?
>
> *Mr Smith:* She has regular features, but you can't call her beautiful. She's too tall and too well-built. Her features are rather irregular, but everyone calls her beautiful. A trifle too short and too slight, perhaps. She teaches singing.
>
> *The clock strikes five.*
>
> *Mrs Smith:* And when are they thinking of getting married, the two of them?

The theatre of the absurd has its roots in the efforts of well-intentioned course designers.

References

1 Richardson S. Letter to Lady Elchin, 22 September 1775. In: Carroll J, editor. *Selected Letters of Samuel Richardson*. Oxford: Clarendon Press; 1964.
2 Wallace P. *Coaching Standardized Patients: for use in the assessment of clinical competence*. New York: Springer; 2006.

3 Cooper JB, Taqueti VR. A brief history of the development of mannequin simulators for clinical education and training. *Qual Saf Health Care.* 2004; **13:** i11–18.

4 Chomsky N. *Aspects of the Theory of Syntax.* Cambridge, MA: MIT Press; 1965.

5 Bellack AA, Kliebard HM, Hyman RT *et al. The Language of the Classroom.* New York: Teachers College Press; 1966.

6 Wittgenstein L. *The Blue and Brown Books.* Oxford: Blackwell; 1958.

7 Wittgenstein L (Anscombe GEM, Rhees R, editors, Anscombe GEM, trans.). *Philosophical Investigations.* Oxford: Blackwell; 1953.

8 Hacker PMS. Wittgenstein. In: Honderich T, editor. *Oxford Companion to Philosophy.* Oxford: Oxford University Press; 1995. pp. 959–63.

9 Hymes D. On communicative competence. In: Pride JB, Holmes J, editors. *Sociolinguistics: selected readings.* Harmondsworth: Penguin; 1972. pp. 269–93.

10 Cohen CJ, Rehnman E. The role of management games in education and research. *Management Sci.* 1961: **7:** 131–66.

11 García Carbonell A, Watts F. Perspectiva histórica de simulación y juego como estrategía docente: de la guerra al aula de lengua para fines específicos. *Ibérica.* 2007; **13:** 65–84.

12 Ricciardi FM, Craft CJ, Malcolm DG *et al. Top Management Decision Simulation: the AMA approach.* American Management Association: New York; 1957.

13 Conan Doyle A. The adventure of the copper beeches. In: *The Return of Sherlock Holmes.* Oxford: Oxford World Classics; 1993 (first published 1892).

14 Greenhalgh T. Narrative-based medicine in an evidence-based world. *BMJ.* 1999; **318:** 323–5.

15 General Medical Council. *Tomorrow's Doctors.* London: General Medical Council; 2003; www.gmc-uk.org/Education/Undergraduate/Tomdoc.Pdf (accessed 10 July 2007).

16 The Bristol Royal Infirmary Enquiry, July 2001; www.bristol-inquiry.org.uk/final_report/report/index.htm (accessed 10 July 2007).

17 Shub D. *Lenin: a biography.* 2nd ed. Harmondsworth: Penguin; 1966. p. 70 (first published 1948).

18 Sayers DL. The lost tools of learning. *National Review,* 19 January 1979, p. 94; www.cambridgestudycenter.com/artilces/Sayers1.htm [sic] (accessed 10 July 2007).

19 Ross EA. Social Control. XIV. Education. *Am J Sociol.* 1900; **5:** 475–87.

20 Dewey J. Science in the course of study. In: *Democracy and Education.* New York: Macmillan; 1916.

21 Gardner H. *Frames of Mind: the theory of multiple intelligences.* London: Heinemann; 1984.

22 Hanna M, Fins JJ. Power and communication: why simulation training ought to be complemented by experiential and humanist learning. *Acad Med.* 2006; **81:** 265–70.

23 Ionesco E (Watson D, trans.). *The Bald Prima Donna. A pseudo-play in one act.* London: Calder; 1958.

CHAPTER 2

A reflection on Socrates

He was 40 years old before he looked in on Geometry; which happened accidentally. Being in a Gentleman's Library, Euclid's Elements lay open, and 'twas the 47 *El. libri* I. He read the Proposition. By G__, sayd he (he would now and then swear an emphaticall Oath by way of emphasis) *this is impossible!* So he read the Demonstration of it, which referred him back to such a Proposition; which proposition he read. That referred him back to another, which he also read. *Et sic deinceps* that at last he was demonstratively convinced of that trueth. This made him in love with Geometry.

(Thomas Hobbes discovers Pythagoras' Theorem,
from *Brief Lives*[1])

Doctors and teachers

From patient-centred medicine to student-centred learning is a short step, and it is the purpose of this chapter and the next to explore the similarities. If we don't understand the similarities between the two, and the fact therefore that we use role play, in a number of respects, to educate doctors to talk like teachers, then we have failed to grasp an important point.

The bridge between the doctor and the teacher is, I would suggest, a kind of democratic, western mindset – a belief in the value of the other person, a desire to take their views seriously and, just as in a democracy all are assumed to have an equal right to their political opinion, a belief that the thoughts of the patient and the student have value. This general view I call 'lay-centredness', and it is to be found in slogans ranging from 'Listen to the patient' to 'The customer is always right.'

There is of course a straightforward danger at the heart of this attitude. There are in fact circumstances under which not everyone's views are equally valid, or equally to be valued. For example, societies set boundaries on freedom of speech. I may legitimately disagree with you about the extent to which a free market is a good thing (in medicine, say), and I may vote accordingly. However, if I seek to argue that certain ethnic groups should have fewer rights than me, few would complain if I was arrested. And when it comes to education and medicine, there are straightforward issues of fact at stake. Compare the following dialogues:

> *Teacher:* How can we help with global warming?
>
> *Pupil:* I think all cars should be banned.
>
> *Teacher:* That's an interesting idea.
>
> *Teacher:* What's the capital of Denmark?
>
> *Pupil:* Berlin.
>
> *Teacher:* That's an interesting idea.

Doctors deal in facts – or rather, a lot of doctors deal in a lot of facts a lot of the time. A great deal of medical training is inevitably concerned with reducing ambiguity, with getting to the kernel of truth at the heart of the baffling evidence. This is the Sherlock Holmes aspect of medicine, as we have seen, which creates a perception of the doctor as solver of puzzles.

From this, it follows that the formal position – the official position for the twenty-first century, as it were – is something like this. Relying on expertise, the doctor sets out the facts. Respecting the patient's rights, the doctor then declares it to be up to the patient what use they want to make of these facts. The role of expertise in professional life, on this basis, is to state facts and their consequences ('Well, you can continue to smoke 50 a day, but you're storing up problems for yourself . . .').

It won't do, of course. One of the many difficulties with patient-centredness is that this absolute demarcation between fact and advice (or at least unsolicited advice) is unsustainable. The previous example is, in the abstract, a statement of fact, just as 'The grass is long' is a statement of fact – smokers develop health problems. However, in context, it surely functions as a piece of advice: 'Stop smoking.' And in any case, as is clear from the fecklessly recalcitrant smoker implied here, there are implications of the choices made which go beyond the patient, to their family, to the costs of treatment of self-inflicted illness, and so on.

Nevertheless, lay-centredness is embedded in modern, western culture, where it may best be considered as the professional simulacrum of democracy. However, certain things follow from this. First, 'patient-centredness' is much less of an original and unique idea than many of its proponents seem to realise. Whether this kind of pause for thought diverts one into a sense that its value is enhanced because it is deeply embedded in our cultural mores, or into a sense that it is therefore part of a twentieth-century bandwagon that is still with us, is a matter of (genuinely) personal choice. However, the depth of its roots in modern thought and modern life cannot be overestimated.

Secondly, simply because it is so culture-bound, it ought to make us wonder about its transferability beyond a western context. This is partly a simple matter of asking whether doctors and patients in other parts of the world might find 'patient-centredness' a helpful way to proceed, if by 'patient-centredness' one means something which can be operationalised as a set of skills. And it should be observed that precisely the debate about whether 'patient-centred medicine' is a good idea is mirrored in an identical debate, couched in identical terms, about 'student-centred education.' In particular, teacher trainees worry about the question of whether the teacher can say 'Well, what do you think?' in response to a question, rather than simply giving the answer, and still maintain appropriate authority, in much the same way as doctors express anxiety about saying 'It's up to you.'

However, this is only part of the debate here. The point to remember about 'patient-centredness' is that it is in large part a concept defined by what it is not. It stands politically and rhetorically as being *not* a set of undesirable qualities. So it is not being mechanistic, not being arrogant, not being patronising, and so on. Perhaps, to an outsider, such statements would resemble nothing so much as the replacement of expertise by vapid attempts at self-analysis and empathy.

These issues have renewed impetus at present because of a growing recognition, echoed as we saw in *Tomorrow's Doctors*, that one thing doctors do with their professional lives is teach:

> In the medical profession, teaching expertise has traditionally been assumed to be a part of clinical or scientific expertise. Only since the second half of the 20th century has teaching been acknowledged as a skill in its own right. Through formal or informal training or supervision of students, junior staff and other professionals, all doctors are involved in teaching to some extent. The presumption that only the proper understanding of a clinical discipline is enough to fulfil a doctor's educational obligation is no longer tenable.[2]

Or, similarly, from an earlier document on the same debate (and notice the almost inevitable cohabitation of buzz-words like 'learner-centred', 'problem solving', 'community setting', 'facilitation' – and, of course, 'communication skills'):

> Changes in undergraduate education have emphasised learner-centred education, problem solving and the acquisition of clinical and communication skills within hospital and community settings. For this reason, more hospital doctors and general practitioners are likely to be involved in teaching and the facilitation of learning, including the provision of feedback about performance, than hitherto.[3]

Teaching responsibility of some sort is in fact a common feature of professional life in general, and in this, too, medicine and the health professions are participating in a wider debate.

I have a straightforward faith in education. I observe that people have learned, and I observe that this has often been in the proximity of competent teachers. I reflect on the good teaching experiences I have had in my own education, and the bad ones I have endured, and I find that highly articulate teachers with imagination, moral depth, wit and enthusiasm have an effect – and that others do, too, but a slower one. I don't want to suggest that only such teachers matter, still less (as I plough grimly from teaching commitment to teaching commitment on, say, a rainy November morning) to claim that I have these qualities myself – but this is how I wish teaching was, and how I would like to portray it, and encourage it to be.

On the status of the expert, or 'A doctor is like a hairdresser'

For two or three years I had my hair cut by a New Zealander whose father wrote language textbooks. This got me thinking.

> *Scene: in the corridor, the Medical School, more or less anywhere*
>
> **A:** Surely a doctor is like anyone else engaged in offering a service to the public. Consider a hairdresser, for example – does such an individual not have expertise, as a doctor has?
>
> **B:** Well, yes, I suppose so. The expertise is less, perhaps, but I see your point. But hairdressing is nothing more than the acquisition of a set of skills – how to handle the scissors, that sort of thing, and you and I wish to believe, my dear alter ego, that medical education involves so much more . . .

A: Indeed we do, but perhaps this is also true for other professional domains. And in any case, as for the idea that hairdressing skills are somehow 'less' than doctoring skills, there is an interesting discussion here. How do you measure and compare relative quantities of skill in different fields? Are the skills of a footballer greater than those of a brain surgeon? A gardener or a headteacher? A painter or a plumber? Is it 'difficulty' that's in question here? And if so, by what yardstick is difficulty measured? But leave that be. The more pertinent issue is to draw your attention to the fact that the hairdresser must, like the doctor, draw on deeper knowledge, a context in which to exercise skills – an understanding of fashion, let's say, a learned or intuitive sense of what cut will suit which person – their looks, their personality, what kind of person they wish to present themselves as. These are deep matters, and . . .

B: You're being facetious . . .

A: Not at all. And, I was going to say, just as one talks all this guff about doctors and their need to communicate with patients, so hairdressers need to present an environment in which their customers feel welcome, feel at home, feel that they are treated as a person of interest even when (the parallel with patients once more, you see) they are less dignified than they would wish – swathed in a gown, with their hair in curlers or one of those peculiar sort of bathing cap affairs that women have their hair pulled through when they're getting it coloured . . .

B: You're blithering . . .

A: I never spoke more truly. An endless ability to talk about your next holiday or the last one, about sport with men, or about boyfriends with women . . .

B: Does the word 'stereotype' mean nothing to you?

A: Merely a matter of recognising familiar patterns, my own dear doppelgänger. And I seem to recall you, pedant that you are, briefly favoured with your custom a hairdresser whose dad had written a standard school textbook for learners of Maori, and how you suddenly enjoyed the ritual of the haircut . . .

B: Touché, I suppose. But I think I've nailed the difference. Your relationship with your hairdresser is purely consumerist. You can go in and say 'Give me the same haircut as . . .' – well, whoever the latest fashionable singer is – and you will have your wish fulfilled, however ill-advised. A doctor must be made of sterner stuff, and not give in to the whims of the addle-headed.

A: Pausing briefly to remark both that you are amusingly unable to name anyone in the public eye below the age of 30, and that the phrase 'latest fashionable singer' is not entirely *au courant* as a use of English, I concede the truth of what you are saying. In your own case, a good hairdresser will sensitively advise you that youth is a stuff which will not endure, and that you model this immutable truth only too well. But in the end, as you imply, you may take umbrage and withdraw your custom. However, you will not do so if a relationship of trust exists, and this is what I have been seeking to assert all along, that . . .

B: Yes, yes, quite. That the communication skills associated with the central task are of less importance than the relationship which underpins them. And that more nebulous concepts such as trust, and the role of the professional as adviser and so on, are of greater significance.

A: Not to say frankly more interesting. Yes, indeed, my point is – if I may abandon my nagging insistence on the analogy with personal grooming – that the difference between the hairdresser and the doctor has to do with the relative weight of their duties and responsibilities. And moreover, although both have areas of expertise, the power and authority of the doctor – power invested in the role not merely by individual patients but by law – is utterly different. The doctor controls access to referrals, to drugs, to treatment, and so on. The difference, I conclude, between the doctor and the hairdresser lies in precisely those areas beyond the boundaries of patient-centredness. The difference, that is, resides in the doctor's right – no, the doctor's duty – to say 'I know better than you. This is not in your best interests.' The very nature of the doctor, the very essence of medical practice, is benign paternalism . . .

B: OK, I get the point.

A: Do you think so, indeed? But I say that you only get the half of it, mon semblable. Because in fact there are details of the analogy with education which I wish to draw more seriously to your attention. And may I just say that this is not the last dialogue the reader will encounter in this chapter.

B: You have, as ever, a hidden agenda, I perceive.

A: No doubt – though the phrase is overused. But such is the inevitable consequence of too much education. At all events, let us talk of Socrates.

Socrates the teacher

If you ask any group of doctors what their worst experience of medical education has been, someone will say 'teaching by humiliation.' This is depressing, because many doctors are in fact excellent teachers, and this is what I want to explore in this chapter. I would argue two things. First, the reason why doctors tend to teach well is that the skills associated with teaching are very similar to those which are typically taught as good consultation skills. Secondly, beyond that, one of the reasons for the similarity is that both consulting and teaching draw on the similar assumptions we have been looking at about what constitutes 'good practice.' In other words, for broad notions of 'patient-centredness' we can substitute no less broad notions of 'student-centredness.'

You could argue that, as with so many other things, the tradition of western education began with the Greeks, and specifically with Socrates, or at any rate with Socrates as we see him through Plato's eyes. Socrates wrote nothing that has come down to us – he exists primarily as the leading figure in the Dialogues written by his pupil, Plato. I follow standard practice in ascribing the methodology pursued in the Dialogues as 'Socratic', although the extent to which it truly arose with Socrates may be unknowable. I should add that, as is probably the case with most people, I want to look at this method as a jumping-off point for thoughts about the way in which teaching skills have developed, and the reader should therefore be aware that I use the term 'teaching skills' fairly loosely.

The methodology itself typically works as follows. Socrates asks a major question, about some abstract term, and then explores the answer he is given with further questions. This kind of often friendly but always pointed cross-examination is known as *elenchus*. The result is that, as we shall see below, an impasse is reached. The original answer to the question is found to lead to a contradiction, a puzzle, a dead end. This is known as an *aporia*. The point of an *aporia* to Socrates is that when it is recognised, it can spur someone on to greater efforts, so that the lazy and unsustainable ideas held at the outset of the conversation are replaced by better or more sophisticated ideas.

The *locus classicus* for Socratic teaching (see also *Language and Clinical Communication* for a little more detail on this passage) arises in the course of the *Meno*,[4] a dialogue between Socrates and one of the rich youths who clustered round him (one of the 'pretty young gentlemen', as Socrates calls them here), seeking knowledge. In the *Meno*, the question being explored is what virtue is.

Meno concludes:

> . . . The thing about 'being good' is that it's different for each of us; it varies according to what we're doing, according to how old we are, and according to our role in life.

('And I imagine, Socrates', he adds rather darkly, 'the same goes for being bad.')

However, this way of looking at things, as Socrates points out, would result merely in a list of virtuous things to do, not – as we would say – in a definition of virtue. Can Meno say what all virtuous actions have in common?

Meno's eventual response, after some toing and froing, is that although, for instance, 'strength' means the same thing regardless of whether one is talking about strength in a man or a woman, a child or an adult, 'Somehow I don't feel it works in quite the same way [with goodness] . . .' (It's one of the virtues – if I can use that word – of Plato's quasi-novelistic style that one can imagine Meno mumbling rather tetchily at this point.) Socrates carries on, leading Meno a merry and complex dance until in the end Meno admits his confusion – the moment of *aporia*:

> Meno: You know, people kept telling me, Socrates, even before I met you, that all you do is go around being baffled by things and baffling everyone else. And now that I've met you, sure enough, I feel as though you're bewitching me, and jinxing me, and casting some strange spell over me, to the point where I'm as baffled as can be. You know what I think? Just to tease you a little – I think you're exactly like that flat-faced numbfish. You certainly look like a numbfish, and you're just the same in other ways as well: because you know what a numbfish does? It makes anyone that gets too close, and touches it, go numb; and that's pretty much what I think you've done to me. My mind and tongue have literally gone numb. I've got no idea how to answer the question. And yet, damn it, I've talked about 'being a good man' *thousands* of times.

(The 'numbfish', or 'torpedo fish', is an electric ray, which gives an electric shock. Socrates' looks were famously unprepossessing, incidentally – hence perhaps Meno's rather personal remarks – in contrast to Meno himself, whose looks draw a number of admiring comments from the philosopher.) Meno's own revealed ignorance disturbs him, and so does the professed ignorance of Socrates, who has a reputation for wisdom. And in this state, asks Meno, where on earth does one start? 'I mean, how can you put before your mind a thing that *you have no knowledge of*, in order to try to find out about it?'

Socrates' answer is spiritual, but it will be clear that we can think of it as educational without betraying him too much. 'Priests and priestesses', he says, '[have made a claim] as beautiful as it [is] true [that] a person's soul can never die.' From which it follows:

> So, since the soul can never die, and has been born over and over again, and has already seen what there is in this world, and what there is in the world beyond – i.e. absolutely everything – there's nothing it hasn't already learned about. So it wouldn't be at all surprising if it managed to remember things, the things it used to know, either about being good or about anything else. Because if the whole of nature is akin, and your soul has already learned and understood everything,

there's no reason why you shouldn't be able, after remembering just *one* thing – most people call it 'learning' – to go on and figure out everything else, as long as you're adventurous and don't get tired of trying to find out about things; in fact, 'finding out about things' and 'learning' are entirely a matter of remembering.

And he then sets out to prove the point, asking Meno to 'Do me a favour and call one of those attendants of yours' – that is, an uneducated slave who we may presume has been hanging around in the background – so that he may teach him, and in so doing demonstrate that the slave *already has* the knowledge that Socrates is concerned with.

So then Socrates draws a square:

> *Socrates:* Tell me, then, boy, do you know what a square is? You know that a square . . . *[He draws a square in the sand with his stick]* . . . looks like this?
>
> *Boy:* Yes.
>
> *Socrates:* So a square is a figure with four sides – these lines here – all the same length?
>
> *Boy:* Of course.

I shall try to draw brief parallels with modern teaching as we go along, but the reader should be very conscious of the risk of anachronism. Socrates and Plato inevitably and frequently sound modern (we are their intellectual heirs, after all), and it is tempting and easy to overstate the case.

Notice here, however, that Socrates – in formal teaching mode at this stage – begins by asking questions, and that his preliminary questions are designed to establish the slave's present level of understanding. (Has he heard the word 'square'? Does he know what a square is?) This is, if I may force the comparison a little, a kind of needs analysis. Questions are, of course, nine-tenths of Socratic dialogue, and in much the same way, teaching – or at any rate teaching of individuals or small groups – is undertaken in precisely the same way in our world.

Socrates then asks the slave to suppose that one side of the square is two feet long. If he draws a cross within his square, the points bisecting each side, would this not produce four smaller squares, each one foot by one foot? From which it is fairly clear that the area of a square two feet by two feet is four square feet, is it not? The slave agrees.

Then, in what seems to me to be one of the most exciting moments in the history of education, Socrates, accidentally or deliberately, leads the boy into making a mistake:

Socrates: . . . Now can you imagine there being another square, also with equal sides, just like this one, but twice the area?

Slave: Yes.

Socrates: So how many square feet would that one be?

Slave: Eight square feet.

This is a common error which any maths teacher will recognise – if you double the length of the lines, from two feet to four feet, then surely you double the area, from four square feet to eight square feet? Not so, of course, and Socrates proceeds as follows:

Socrates: All right, now listen: try and tell me how long each *side* of that one would have to be. Look – each side of this one here is two feet long. What about each side of a square that's twice the area?

Slave: That's obvious, Socrates: twice as long.

Socrates: You see, Meno? I'm not teaching him anything. All I'm doing is asking questions. And now he thinks he knows which line will get us an area of eight square feet. Doesn't he?

Meno: Yes, he does.

Socrates: So does he know?

Meno: He certainly doesn't.

So Socrates continues with his questions, drawing on the sand as he goes along, enjoining Meno and the other spectators (and we can include ourselves here) to 'watch him as he remembers, step by step, the way remembering should be done.' He demonstrates that you don't get an answer of eight square feet if the sides of the square are two feet long, nor four feet long, nor finally three feet long. So what length do you need? To which the answer is:

Slave: Honest to God, Socrates, I don't know.

Once more, this is the moment of *aporia*, the instant when a misconception lies exposed for what it is. The slave is 'baffled', he feels 'numb', just as Meno did earlier. And, says Socrates (in a phrase which many more cynical teachers might consider demonstrates an undue faith in the power of motivation), 'now he'll be happy to try and find out what he doesn't know.'

Socrates then goes back to the original square, two feet by two feet, and adds another square of the same size below it, and then another beside it, as follows:

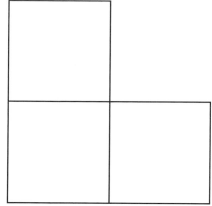

FIGURE 2.1

From this, it is clear to the slave that the addition of a fourth square (in the top right), again two feet by two feet, would give a larger square which is 'four times the area', not two.

So, then, how does one arrive at a square which is eight square feet?

Socrates proceeds to elicit from the boy the possibility of starting off with a square which is four feet by four feet, bisecting each side and joining up the four bisection points (*see* Figure 2.2), so creating a square inside the larger square which is demonstrably half the size – he just needs to count the number of triangles in the larger square (8) and compare this with the number which go to make up the diamond within it (4). The diamond is therefore eight square feet.

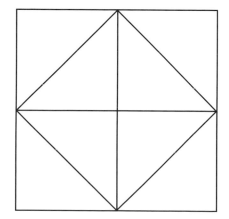

FIGURE 2.2

(This way of doing the mathematics, as has been pointed out by Cooke,[5] approaches a version of Pythagoras' theorem. Pythagoras' contribution was to understand the general principles behind the theorem, and to begin to appreciate its power.)

And Socrates concludes:

> *Socrates:* . . . inside someone with no knowledge (of whatever it might be) there are correct opinions about the things he doesn't know?
>
> *Meno:* So it seems.
>
> *Socrates:* And although right now he'll find these opinions are hazy and dreamlike . . . if you ask him the same questions over and over again, and in lots of different ways, you can be sure that he'd end up knowing about these things as precisely as anyone?
>
> *Meno:* Yes, he probably would.

And there we are.

What relevant conclusions can we draw from this? Certainly, that questions and answers are the engine which makes teaching happen. But let's try and go rather further.

We don't have to believe in reincarnation, or the immortality of the soul, to recognise that good teaching consists partly of recollecting, in the modern sense of the word (that is, recollections from the present life rather than a previous one). This is why teachers begin by reminding their class of what took place in the last lesson – by re-orientating them towards the subject area. Nor is it hard to recognise the role of 'elicitation' in education (note the phrase translated above as 'eliciting or as men say learning'). The essence of learner-centredness, in other words, is that learning comes from within.

One of the most interesting things is that the slave uses his previous knowledge wrongly, and gets something wrong. It is the possibility of making a mistake as a result of forming a wrong hypothesis (in this case, that by doubling the length of the side of a square you double its area) which demonstrates that we don't learn simply by repeating things parrot-fashion. Rather, our brain tries to make sense of what is new by fitting it into patterns we already have.

Patterns laid down in a previous life, Plato might want to argue. In more modern (but not necessarily less contentious) terms once more, patterns which are part of our experience or of the innate capacities with which we were born.

The question of whether we have innate ideas, in the philosophers' phrase, or merely some kind of predisposition to organise experience, or whether we are born with a *tabula rasa* – an empty page on which experience writes as we go along – has turned up in many guises over the centuries, most recently directly and indirectly through the debate between Skinner and Chomsky and its aftermath (see *Language and Clinical Communication*). What matters here is that clearly we all, if we are members of *Homo sapiens* with normal function, have something which predisposes us to make sense of the world by finding patterns, and it is this aspect of our being into which teaching taps.

Finally, as we have seen, the slave is taken to the verge of an apprehension of the great Pythagorean theorem. In other words, he is transformed from being a complete nobody ('Is he Greek at least? Does he speak Greek?' are, tellingly, Socrates' first questions of Meno, before he begins talking to him directly) to a nascent mathematician in one lesson. The richness of the context is extraordinary – here is the kernel of a whole way of looking at the world, a universe of mathematical rigour, of elegant and simple truth, set out in the sand for an untutored youth. This is what education, focussed on the learner, can do.

References

1 Aubrey J. Thomas Hobbes. In: Dick OL, editor. *Brief Lives.* London: Martin, Secker and Warburg; 1949 (written *c.*1679–97). p. 150.

2 British Medical Association. *Doctors as Teachers.* London: British Medical Association; 2006; http://web.bma.org.uk/ap.nsf/AttachmentsByTitle/PDFdoctorsasteachers/$FILE/Doctorsasteachers.pdf (accessed 31 January 2007).

3 General Medical Council. *The Doctor as Teacher.* London: General Medical Council; 1999; www.gmcuk.org/education/publications/doctor_as_teacher.asp (accessed 31 January 2007).

4 Plato (Beresford A, trans.). *Meno.* Harmondsworth: Penguin; 2005 (written *c.*380 BC). Jowett translation available online at http://classics.mit.edu/Plato/meno.html (accessed 23 October 2007).

5 Cooke R. *The History of Mathematics: a brief course.* 2nd ed. Hoboken, NJ: Wiley-Interscience; 2005.

CHAPTER 3

The language of the classroom

In the penumbra of their attention most teachers have a kind of concern for language. It may be a desperate sense that their pupils' pitiful gropings for words and their botching together of a few tortured written sentences reduce their language to an absurd caricature. Or they may feel in a way which is rarely explicit that there are linguistic proprieties which belong with a subject for which they have a responsibility. More shadowy still is a sense that some kind of spoken contribution by pupils helps them to learn.

(Harold Rosen, *Towards a Language Policy Across the Curriculum*[1]).

Socrates in education

So far as Socrates is concerned, what we primarily observe in him is the idea that truth is sought rather than found. And that education involves reflection and self-understanding ('Know yourself', he famously said and, almost as famously, 'The unexamined life is not worth living'). We learn by introspection, and also by the study of our errors, and a recognition of our ignorance. And we observe in Socrates, too, that the teacher's fundamental resource is the deployment of questions in an unending dialogue, not the supply of answers from a reservoir of expertise.

Of course – to stress this point again – this is a careful selection from Socratic thought and methodology which in more recent times can be traced from the general ethos of Renaissance education through to Rousseau and the rise of the Constructivist movement in the USA, associated principally with

Dewey and the cluster of great educationalists working in that environment and that era. (There is a very extensive literature on Constructivist education. Brophy[2] gives the general flavour of the contemporary position, while Williams and Burden[3] offer a straightforward account of the psychological background.)

The idea of Constructivism is, in essence, that by reflecting on our experience we construct a model of how the world is. 'Reality' is, in this sense, an internal and subjective construct. This does not mean, of course, that we are typically at risk of reaching perverse or capricious views about the nature of the world in which we have our being, because we are capable of rational understanding (although see Chapter 8 for some remarks on the dangers of the kind of relativism to which a constructivist view may give rise).

At the heart of the Constructivist movement is what we now call, in a kind of shorthand, 'learner-centredness.' This was not, I hasten to add, a phrase that was used in quite its modern guise at the time, although Dewey routinely speaks of 'begin[ing] with the experience of the learner.'[4] Indeed, as Garrison and Neiman suggest,[5] there is a 'common error' associated with the name of Dewey:

> Dewey did not believe in 'student-centered teaching' if that means 'let the child do what it wants.' Indeed, Dewey wrote *Experience and Education* to correct the excess of 'progressivism''s misinterpretation of his work.

However, although Dewey and his colleagues tend not to talk about the minutiae of classroom management or classroom language, the philosophical underpinning is democratic, liberal, and in many senses a mirror image of the young USA. In this respect, though, it should be noted in passing that some educationalists[6] would point to the question–answer sequence of Socratic and subsequent thinking and the 'gentle inquisitions'[7] of the modern classroom, and wonder about the passivity of it all, as we shall see. This, nevertheless, is essentially Dewey's vision:[8]

> A democracy is more than a form of government; it is primarily a mode of associated living, of conjoint communicated experience. The extension in space of the number of individuals who participate in an interest so that each has to refer his own action to that of others, and to consider the action of others to give point and direction to his own, is equivalent to breaking down barriers of class, race and national territory which kept men from perceiving the full import of their activity.

It is at this time (around the turn of the twentieth century), too, that the first stirrings of what we have since learned to summarise as 'patient-centredness' can be identified. Behind much of this is the great Osler's dictum, cited in various different forms, along the lines of 'Listen to your patient: he will tell you the diagnosis', a version at one level of the modern view that most diagnoses can be reached on the basis of history taking alone, but with the added point that what Osler was talking about here was not *taking* a history but *listening* to one. He is probably nearer to contemporary ideas of narrative-based medicine than anything else. That is to say, it is the patient's words that count – and not only the diagnosis but also its meaning which shine through.

What we are looking at is not the simultaneous, coincidental rise of a patient-centred and a student-centred world, but two versions of the same movement, wearing different professional garb, and reflecting a consensus about the nature of professional interaction. It is a shared view that we ought to live and work and undertake professional transactions in a world which is lay-centred. This is in effect the western, liberal consensus about professional life, and in that sense a reflection in miniature of the broad socio-political consensus that is taken for granted in some parts of the world, but not all. Tolerant, considerate, willing to listen to the point of view of others, and so on – this is how the west likes to see itself, free from political authoritarianism. In education free from formality, free from pronouncements about how the world is – free to think, free to challenge. And in the clinic, free to enter into equal discussion rather than, in the old phrase, following doctor's orders. As I say – the way we want to be thought of.

Perhaps the single most influential exponent of lay-centredness was Carl Rogers, the great psychotherapist and humanist, whose *Client-Centred Therapy*,[9] (he also uses the term 'student therapy' here – 'client-centredness' later transmutes into 'person-centredness') had considerable influence through the 1950s and beyond. Rogers has had considerable influence on medicine, or at any rate on the discursive specialties such as psychiatry and primary care. However, he is very highly regarded generally as an educator, principally because his lay-centredness both echoed and helped to develop ideas whose hour had come in any case, and also through his belief in experiential learning – a doctrine which he developed, and in which he invested a huge amount of emotional as well as rational capital:

> Experience is, for me, the highest authority. The touchstone of validity is my own experience. No other person's ideas, and none of my own ideas, are as authoritative as my experience. It is to experience that I must return again and again, to discover a closer approximation to truth as it is in the process of becoming in me. Neither the Bible nor the prophets – neither Freud nor research

– neither the revelations of God nor man – can take precedence over my own direct experience. My experience is not authoritative because it is infallible. It is the basis of authority because it can always be checked in new primary ways. In this way its frequent error or fallibility is always open to correction.[10]

This famous quotation is revealing in all sorts of ways. It demonstrates very clearly Rogers' own roots in religion – he was brought up in a religious family, and at one time expected to go into the ministry. Indeed in one of his central beliefs – that the therapist should have 'unconditional personal regard' for the client (just as the parent should have for the child) – there are fairly straightforward echoes of a Christian *agape*, a love and acceptance of others, a willingness to love the sinner and hate the sin. Equally, that claim for personal 'authority' looks a little like a rejection of the *auctoritas* of the church, a rejection of the right of others to say what is or ought to be the case – which in turn is a version of authority which applies equally well to religion or to education.

Looking inwards in order to learn is, of course, not unlike Socrates' ideas of learning through recollection or, as I suggest above, through the process of filtering new information through one's past experience. However, it would be unwise to make too much of this, given the difference in time and background. Nevertheless, so far as education is concerned, Rogers distinguishes between 'cognitive' and 'experiential' learning. The former, which includes such elements of rote learning as reciting multiplication tables, is unsurprisingly disparaged in favour of the latter.

Putting it this way makes Rogers seem like a thoroughgoing moral and for that matter educational relativist – of the kind who would, as it were, value whatever the student says because, hey, your views are as good as mine. This is indeed the kind of criticism that has been levelled at him, and it is aspects of his work, poorly studied and understood, which were part of the educational free-for-all of a certain kind of classroom a generation ago – the type characterised, to pick up that phrase again, as 'let[ting] the child do what it wants.' Perhaps one of Rogers' most endearing qualities, or for some one of his great weaknesses, is his optimism about humanity, his belief that to value the experience of others, and by extension their ability to make sense of their own experiences, is indeed to help them learn.

Another formulation of the central relationship between what we learn and the world beyond us is that of Piaget. Originally a biologist, Piaget began to study what he termed 'genetic epistemology', roughly defined as the study of how thought takes place in the process of development. He saw this as a process of 'adaptation', consisting of two components. The first is *assimilation* of new information into an existing state of understanding – for example, a child may learn the hard way that a sensation of heat can be linked to getting burned, and will therefore build up a sense of the general pattern (a 'schema') that heat and burning are associated. The other central process of adaptation is *accommodation*, where we discover that our existing schemata do not fit the facts, and we have to alter our understanding in order to take account of this. For example, a child may have a schema that cats like to be picked up, because the family pet accepts this with a good grace – but they may discover subsequently that this is not true of all cats.

The pattern-building process of assimilation is central to our ability as adults to make sense of the world without thinking everything through from first principles. If I see a large, grey, indistinct shape in the middle distance while out on safari I might postulate an elephant. If I peer up at the sky from my office window I am presumably more likely to guess at a cloud. Without these patterns we are stuck, and will not be able to function. However, to rely on them too much is to run the danger of stereotyping. Note here how Dewey's vision of democracy, quoted above, can be understood in just these terms – of reaching out to others through just this process of mutual accommodation, of 'us' to 'them' and 'them' to 'us.'

All of this gives us an image of perfect classroom learning. One can imagine a situation where advances are made through discussion, moving from one state of understanding to the next, although all such states are provisional and all are therefore subject to future changes in the light of new experiences and our willingness to accommodate them. To value the learner's views, under this kind of system, is to value the learner's potential for understanding, to take seriously their provisional comments (recognising that our understanding is no less provisional), but subjecting them to scrutiny just as we may expect our own views to be subjected to scrutiny. All of which, we might agree, was essentially the Socratic ideal in the first place.

This is unquestionably attractive as a view. However, the considerable difficulties involved need to be faced. For example, Socrates never seems to lose an argument. Why not? Well, for structural reasons, as Plato's mouthpiece, it would be inconvenient – but there are other considerations, too. We are clearly to think of him as someone who has a more sophisticated mind – he understands the processes of abstract reasoning better than anyone else. And, for all that Socrates claimed to be wise only in that he at least knew he was ignorant, in the end it is pretty obvious that he 'knows more' in some real sense than anyone else. And, even at the purely psychological level, Socrates is in charge. He leads the argument, and the young men around him are deferential. Socrates takes the lead in the language of the classrooms that he manages.

This is the conundrum of lay-centredness again. Socrates is the expert, just as the doctor in practice is the expert. There is no point in turning away from this central fact. Teachers and students may at times (not often enough, perhaps) have the opportunity for exploratory debate – doctors and patients may also have just such an opportunity. However, for much of the time, the student and the patient alike must deal not with provisionals but with what, by agreement, they take to be facts. What is two plus two? What is the capital of Denmark? How will my hypertension affect my lifestyle?

And, to finish with a rhetorical question, who knows the answer? Not the lay person, or the meeting is a waste of time. It is the expert who knows.

The contract of engagement

In all interactions there are rules of the game. The hairdresser has no right to swear at me, nor do I have the right to be rude to her, and so on. As a patient I have a right to suppose that the doctor will treat me with appropriate levels of courtesy, respect, and so on. However, beyond the point at which language use serves to identify social roles and foster social relationships, there are other things as well, perhaps in all forms of service encounters, and certainly, in a very crucial way, in both medicine and teaching.

Teachers and doctors have, as we would all accept, ethical obligations to their charges. For example, they must seek to identify and act in the lay person's best interests. Equally, the lay participant also has obligations, and this is less certainly handled in the literature. It is clear enough in the classroom, where there will be a formal way of addressing a failure to meet these obligations, which will then become labelled 'bad behaviour' and addressed through sanctions.

In the surgery, the position is more complex. Doctors of course have rights with regard to patients – as a final sanction they may choose not to see someone who is violent, disruptive or insulting. However, just as a great deal of classroom 'bad behaviour' has its roots in something other than a desire to disrupt for the sake of it, so patients who are not good at being patients are often unaware of their problems. For example, Towle and colleagues[11] suggest the following as a 'preliminary list' of desirable 'patient competencies':

1 define (for oneself) the preferred doctor–patient relationship
2 find a physician and establish, develop and adapt a partnership
3 articulate (for oneself) health problems, feelings, beliefs and expectations in an objective and systematic manner
4 communicate with the physician in order to understand and share relevant information (such as that from competency 3) clearly and at the appropriate time in the medical interview

5   access information
6   evaluate information
7   negotiate decisions, give feedback, resolve conflict and agree on an action
    plan.

It will be seen that this is itself a set of competencies designed in a fairly abstract way – or, given the context, perhaps 'fairly holistic' is a better term. And behind the competencies, I would suggest, it's fairly easy to see that what is required is what one might call a responsible approach to the consultation. Indeed, as the echoes of the corresponding doctor competencies are obvious enough, what matters is precisely what would, in other circumstances, be called a degree of professionalism.

Towle and colleagues are specifically addressing the concept of shared decision making (SDM) (the reader is also referred to the subsequent *British Medical Journal* report[12]). This is at the heart of contemporary thinking about what the good consultation includes, but it is worth mentioning that the phrase has meaning within education, too, where it tends to be a matter of promoting community inclusion, of getting parents, teachers below management level and others involved in the decision-making processes of a school. In this environment – although it will be clear that the term is being used to mean a different thing – it has been suggested that SDM tends to result in a focus on trivial decisions (on the allocation of parking, or the like), and that trying to adopt new roles and relationships is difficult and uncomfortable.[13]

The same is likely to be true within medicine. There is, at any rate, disquiet about the extent to which SDM actually happens. The finding of one study,[14] published in 1997, that 'Important clinical decisions were common but were rarely preceded by substantive discussion', is probably one that would still be widely accepted.

There is a great deal of recent work on SDM and related matters,[15] and on how to identify and measure it,[16] but I would like at this stage to consider the social contract of the classroom in action, and look at *classroom language research*. This will, I hope, return us to the opening point of this chapter, namely why it is that doctors often make excellent teachers.

Classroom language research

The great educationalists of the early twentieth century had very little to say about classroom management, or about the details of what happens in a classroom – the ebb and flow of discussion in a postgraduate seminar, the mechanics of maintaining discipline and giving instructions with children, the way that information is presented, elicited and tested. None of this was explored in detail until the 1960s, although there is the odd foray earlier than that, such as Romiett Stevens' study published in 1912.[17] (For the interested reader, Brueckner discusses some of these pioneering studies.[18]) For Stevens' study, a group of stenographers were sent into high-school classrooms in New York to try to capture what took place. Stevens believed in the value of noting 'without comment or criticism' exactly what happened in a lesson, as a resource for teacher education. She found that 80% of a teacher's time was taken up with asking questions. However, finding this out was difficult:[19]

> Even some of our most expert reporters have been put to rout when called upon to use such terms as simultaneous linear equation, abscissa, ordinate, x-axis in one hour, and Praxiteles, Thucydides, Phidias, Xenophon in the next. This difficulty is further augmented by the fact of the almost universal custom of high-school pupils to speak indistinctly, to pronounce words carelessly, or to trail off their sentences into nothingness.

And this was the rub. An accurate record was beyond the available technology and the ingenuity of the stenographers, and so it remained for another half century or so (it remains one of the great advantages of studying communication in the clinic or surgery that the data are unusually easy to transcribe). One clever solution, which I mention here because the basic technique is so useful, was developed in the 1960s, and became a widely used way of approaching the study of classroom language, and of giving advice to teachers. It has occasionally been used in a clinical setting as well.[20] This was Ned Flanders' Interactive Analysis System (FIAS).[21] (Alas, 'Ned Flanders' is an unfortunate name since the advent of *The Simpsons*.) Flanders proposed 10 categories (*see* Table 3.1) as covering all that might happen in the classroom. The idea was that every three seconds the observer should place a cross against the activity which corresponded to what appeared to be happening. This meant that after three minutes, for example, one would have a string of 60 crosses which could be joined up to give typical patterns. I should add that it is extremely easy to train oneself to do this, simply by counting 'one two three' internally.

It's also an excellent methodology to use, pre-theoretically, for other aspects of teaching. For example, consider viva exams. One might be concerned to note the extent to which the examiner was talking, the extent to which the student was talking, and also the extent to which the examiner was, say, asking for more detail or offering encouragement. It's very easy to set up just these four categories, and to look at the pattern which emerges. Table 3.2 gives a real example, where 'EQ' is 'examiner question', 'SR' is 'student response',

'EC' is 'examiner asks for more detail or clarification', and 'EA' is 'examiner acknowledges or encourages.'

Table 3.1 Flanders' interaction analysis categories (FIAC)

Teacher talk	Response	1 Accepts feeling
		2 Praises or encourages
		3 Accepts or uses ideas of pupils
		4 Asks questions
	Initiation	5 Lecturing
		6 Giving directions
		7 Criticising or justifying authority
Pupil talk	Response	8 Pupil talk – response
	Initiation	9 Pupil talk – initiation
Silence		10 Silence or confusion

Table 3.2 Modified FIAC in action

EQ	xx		xxx			
SR	xx xxxx xx xxx		xxxx xxxxx xx		xxxxx	
EC				x		
EA	xx x x			x	x x	

This shows the first two minutes of a viva. There is a clear general pattern emerging, and one which allows us to draw a few tentative conclusions. The balance of speaking – 27 crosses against the student, 13 crosses against the examiner – is encouraging, and suggests that the examiner is allowing plenty of opportunity for the student to demonstrate their knowledge. The frequency but apparent brevity of the EA category implies a supportive examiner, but not one who interrupts. The lack of requests for clarification under EC may imply a good student, who doesn't need prompting, and so on.

I've taken this example because it seems – at least to me – perfectly straightforward to say that this is how viva stations ought to be handled. However, firstly, it is much less easy to be sure about what constitutes 'good practice' in some more global sense, and secondly, it is clear that desirable categories might well change depending on the activity. A viva, fairly obviously, ought to differ from teaching in the sense that the teacher cannot really offer evaluation, and the positive reinforcement on offer will be different – low-key reassurance that the student is working along the right lines, rather than full-scale enthusiastic endorsement.

The other point which is I think is particularly noticeable is that the categories on offer are not unlike the kind of things that are often quoted as good consultation practice, and it is easy to see how they might be adapted. In other words, both disciplines have measures of power.

Classroom language research (CLR) has been a burgeoning industry for the last 30 years, following through a variety of approaches. At a structural level, Sinclair and Coulthard's classic study from the mid-1970s[22] has been extremely influential. The aim of this approach was, in essence, to build up a picture of how one could analyse units of language longer than a sentence (once more, there don't seem to be 'rules' for this in the way that there are 'rules' for grammar – merely tendencies), and the choice of the classroom setting was initially secondary level. The authors identified a common pattern, known as the 'IRF sequence' (or, more recently, 'IRE'), standing for Initiation, Response and Feedback (or Evaluation), respectively. Let us return to a version of our previous example to stand as an archetype:

> *Teacher (Initiation):* What's the capital of Denmark?
>
> *Pupil (Response):* Copenhagen.
>
> *Teacher (Evaluation):* Good.

Or alternatively:

> *Teacher (Initiation):* What's the capital of Denmark?
>
> *Pupil (Response):* Berlin.
>
> *Teacher (Evaluation):* Hmm. Are you sure?

This is the way that a great deal of teaching operates.

Real examples are of course much more complex – full of wrong turnings, moments of confusion, and stray noises off. In this example, the IRE sequence remains clear enough, but less obvious than in the archetype:[23]

> *Teacher:* Tell us more about that. Who told them to go to a private school?
>
> *Jamie:* (Inaudible) Kicked them out and expelled them.
>
> *Teacher:* Who did that to them? According to what you read in the story, who did that?
>
> *Students:* (Chorus) Teachers. Parents. Courts.

Teacher: I got teachers, parents, courts . . . Did everybody read the same story here? Pensie?

Pensie: From the school . . .

Teacher: A school. Pensie was correct. I think she was looking for . . .

Sinclair and Coulthard's *Towards an Analysis of Discourse*[22] lends itself very well to teacher-training courses, where versions of the methodology have been widely used, at least in the UK – and above all it seems to lend itself well to studies of power in the classroom. This, interestingly, is what was picked up at the time, and over the years the same quantifiable measures have been used to explore aspects of power in both teaching and the consultation – for example, percentage of words spoken by the lay participant, number and percentage of occasions on which the lay participant initiates the topic for conversation, the length of turn of both parties (i.e. how long they talk before the other person begins to do so), and so on. 'Student-centredness', in other words, is discussed in terms not dissimilar to the way in which 'patient-centredness' is discussed.

The consultation also often has an IRE sequence:

I: What's brought you here today?

R: I keep getting these dreadful headaches.

E: Oh dear.

I: And can you show me where you get them?

R: Well, it's like someone's put a band round my head.

E: Right.

This is invented data. As we have seen, a real transcript is of course more confusing, but the elements of Initiation (i.e. question), Response (i.e. answer) and Evaluation (here the doctor's accepting but neutral 'hmm', etc.) are fairly clear in the example below. (For transcription conventions, *see* Appendix.)

D: And in the mean time can you tell me, when you get this sort of feeling, how long would it stay with you for is it the sort of feeling that lasts for weeks or months?

P: No, it might stop for about maybe a week or fortnight, three weeks/you know and/

D: /Hmm hmm hmm hmm/when was the last time you had it?

P: Oh it's I think it's about twelve months maybe

D: Maybe?

P: Hmm.

D: OK/

P: /Might be a little I'm not quite/sure now

D: /Yeh

P: Erm, I know I had one down at the the other house where we lived/and then I had to come down and see I seen/the other doctor about it you know

D: /Hmm hmm/oh yeh

P: But it just comes on all of a sudden

D: Yeh. Have/you had any recent upsets that might have set it off?//

P: /You know//No.

D: No.

P: No.

D: Any recent/stresses that might have set it off?//

P: /the//the only thing what might be fetching it on, I'm going abroad in four weeks' time.

D: Hmm hmm.

This kind of structural approach revealed fairly clearly the extent to which teacher language was concerned – or seemed to be concerned – with control. The kind of study that Sinclair and Coulthard initiated gave rise to discussions very similar to those in medical education – having described what did happen, could one prescribe what ought to happen? And, as in medical education, the answer remains unclear, and for very similar reasons.

This has been no more than a sketch of enormously complex issues. What I conclude is this. There is a cloud of ideas which hovers around our daily life concerning how we want to live, how we want to sustain relationships with each other, and how we want to conduct our public business as learners, teachers, patients, clinicians, consumers, customers – in every public role that we have. These ideas seem to me to be political and cultural at heart, and to deserve treatment at that level. And 'patient-centredness' is no more and no less than the local enactment of these preconceptions, the local answer to the question 'What do we value?'

This means, I would argue, that there is a sense in which 'patient-centredness' is an illusion, in the way that answers to all vast questions such as Meno's 'What is virtue?' are illusory.

Finally, one of the central issues in the study of classroom language is the nature of *authenticity*. The most famous single example of this, long recognised (see, however, a good recent discussion by van Lier[24]), is the strange way in which questions are handled in the IRE sequence. In other words, think how odd it would be to be standing on the street and participating in the following dialogue:

> A: Excuse me, where's the nearest bank?

> B: Just round the corner on your left.

> A: Correct.

The language of the classroom is not the language of the world. Teacher language consists of questions to which the answer is, by and large, already known.

References

1 Rosen H. Towards a language policy across the curriculum. In: Barnes D, Britton J, Rosen H, editors. *Language, the Learner and the School*. Harmondsworth: Penguin; 1969.

2 Brophy J, editor. *Social Constructivist Teaching: affordances and constraints*. Oxford: Elsevier; 2002.

3 Williams M, Burden RL. *Psychology for Language Teachers: a social constructivist approach*. Cambridge: Cambridge University Press; 1997.

4 Dewey J. Science in the course of study. In: *Democracy and Education*. New York: Macmillan; 1916. Available online at http://books.google.co.uk/ (accessed 25 October 2007).

5 Garrison J, Neiman A. Pragmatism and education. In: Blake N, Smeyers P, Smith R, Standish P, editors. *The Blackwell Guide to the Philosophy of Education*. Malden, MA: Blackwell; 2003. p. 29.

6 Mehan H. The role of discourse in learning, schooling, and reform. In: McLeod B, editor. *Language and Learning: educating linguistically diverse students*. Albany, NY: State University of New York Press; 1994. pp. 71–96.

7 Eeds M, Wells D. Grand conversations: an exploration of meaning construction in literature study groups. *Res Teaching English*. 1989; **23**: 4–29.

8 Dewey J. Individuality, equality and superiority. In: Boydston JA, editor. *John Dewey: the middle works. Volume 13.* Carbondale, IL: Southern Illinois University Press; 1922/1983: pp. 295–300.

9 Rogers C. *Client-Centred Therapy: its current practice, theory and implications.* London: Constable; 1951.

10 Rogers C. *On Becoming a Person: a therapist's view of psychotherapy.* London: Constable; 1961.

11 Towle A, Godolphin W, Richardson A. *Competencies for Informed Shared Decision-Making (ISDM): report on interviews with physicians, patients and patient educators and focus group meetings with patients.* Vancouver: University of British Columbia; 1997.

12 Towle A, Godolphin W. Framework for teaching and learning informed shared decision making. *BMJ.* 1999; **319**: 766–71.

13 Lashway L. The limits of shared decision-making. *ERIC Digest.* 1996; **108**.

14 Braddock CH, Fihn SD, Levinson W *et al.* How doctors and patients discuss routine clinical decisions. *J Gen Intern Med.* 1997; **12**: 339–45.

15 Edwards A, Elwyn G, editors. *Evidence-Based Patient Choice: inevitable or impossible?* Oxford: Oxford University Press; 2001.

16 Elwyn G, Edwards A, Mowle S *et al.* Measuring the involvement of patients in shared decision making: a systematic review of instruments. *Patient Educ Counsel.* 2001; **1406**: 1–19.

17 Stevens R. *The Question as a Means of Efficiency in Instruction: a critical study of classroom practice.* New York: Teachers College, Columbia University; 1912.

18 Brueckner LJ. Diagnostic analysis of classroom procedures. *Elementary School J.* 1926; **1**: 25–40; www.jstor.org

19 Stenographic Reports of High School Lessons: high school lessons. *Teachers College Record.* 1910; **11**: 1; www.tcrecord.org (accessed 27 April 2006).

20 Kishi K. Communication patterns of health teaching and information recall. *Nurs Res.* 1983; **32**: 230–5.

21 Flanders NA. *Analyzing Teaching Behavior.* Reading, MA: Addison-Wesley; 1970.

22 Sinclair JM, Coulthard M. *Towards an Analysis of Discourse: the English used by teachers and pupils.* London: Longman; 1975.

23 Tharp R, Gallimore R. *Rousing Minds to Life.* Cambridge: Cambridge University Press; 1988.

24 van Lier L. *Interaction in the Language Curriculum: awareness, autonomy and authenticity.* London: Longman; 1996.

CHAPTER 4

Rich contexts

Dramatise it! Dramatise it!

(Henry James, *The Art of the Novel*[1])

Introduction

Meanings arise from context. This is what the image of the king's move tells us. And it is precisely the relationship between an abstract concept and its meaning in the world which Henry James is thinking of in his repeated exhortations to himself and others to 'dramatise' ideas. In just the same way, the doctor's understanding of a particular set of symptoms deepens as it is enriched by a lifetime's experience, by the process of gathering in a lifetime's worth of contexts. In this sense, 'meanings' are inexhaustible.

The same point can be made in another way, by thinking in curriculum terms, thinking that is of the distinction between deductive and inductive approaches. The former begins with the lecture – generalised statements delivered *ex cathedra*. The latter begins with the kinds of methodology associated with PBL and, more broadly, any kind of learning that focuses on the achievement of tasks centred on a single case. Such cases, scenarios, problems or tasks – whatever label is used – are potentially infinite in their reach. In this respect, beginning with a single scenario is like searching on the Internet, looking for an answer to a single question. You might begin by searching for something as mundane as a support group for people with depression, and before you notice the time, midnight has come and gone and you're finding out more than you ever needed to know about the planet Saturn.

In this chapter and the next one I have tried to unpick three scenarios, in order to show a few (but only a few) of the directions in which such things can be taken. You will, I hope, be able to think of many other possibilities – and this is the whole point. There are no limits to this kind of work.

To repeat, however, I don't claim great originality for the type of activity suggested. Rather I have tried to open up for discussion some of the techniques that are in fairly common use. Also, in the interests of space, and because the relevant advice changes with time and place, I have not gone into detail here or in subsequent chapters about how to follow up such teaching – the possibility of support groups, helpful Internet sites, patient information leaflets and so on, nor have I discussed the basic reading around the clinical areas which might be appropriate. And, finally, I have chosen to look simply at role-play activity, rather than the full range of types of simulation – for example, the virtual environments discussed by Smith and colleagues[2] in their proposals for 'PCL' (patient-centred learning). What follows, then, is the bread and butter of role-play activity, namely scenarios treated as self-standing events.

All three scenarios have a primary care setting, as this is the setting with which I am most familiar. However, the setting is irrelevant. The principles are the same irrespective of the details, and the overarching instructions for the reader working in a different setting would be simply as follows:

- For the first scenario, think of a common source of conflict between a patient and a health professional.
- For the second scenario, think of a patient who cannot understand what a polite refusal is, and put him or her in a situation with a health professional.
- For the third scenario, place a colleague in a dilemma which can be resolved by asking a fellow health professional to do something unethical.

All three of these scenarios involve people who do not play by the rules of the game, in different ways. The first, as we shall see, cannot do so because he is momentarily in the grip of anger and distress. In the second scenario the person has a long-term problem – an inability to understand the nuances of what people say to her, which may partly be the cause or the consequence of the obvious, longer-term unhappiness she displays. And in the third scenario the person knows the rules, but chooses not to play by them.

These scenarios form the basis – again, this is the point – of lessons which may be very short (20 minutes) or very long (an hour or more), depending on how much time is available. I ought to stress that we have almost never had the luxury of longer periods of time for single scenarios, or for working with and following up the detailed notes, because of the way in which our curriculum is structured. Nevertheless, for the first two of these scenarios, I have included a fully written up set of scenario notes, which can be given to participants at the close of the lesson.

Note incidentally that in this chapter and the following ones, where I look at role-play lessons in detail, I use the terms 'participant', 'facilitator' and 'role player' as the most neutral available.

Rich context scenario 1: Dealing with anger

Participant notes

Your next patient is Mr Oliver Stafford. He is generally well, and there is no indication of why he is here today.

You know Mr Stafford and his family slightly. His wife is called Hilary, and both of them are teachers. They have one son, Thomas, aged 5. All of them are patients at the practice.

From memory, you saw <u>Mrs</u> Stafford with Thomas last week. Thomas was brought to see you with an 18-hour history of diarrhoea, diffuse central stomach ache and anorexia. After examination, you decided that this was probably a viral illness, and advised fluids only for 24 hours and rest. You also told Mrs Stafford to contact you if the pain worsened – she didn't. Your computer entry reads '*Viral gastroenteritis. Advise plenty of fluids; no food for 24 hours; contact GP if condition worsens.*'

The notes made at Thomas' last visit were as follows:

'*D&V. Abdo NAD. Prob viral. Fluids. Starve 24 hrs. See if worsens.*'

'Dealing with anger': lesson plan

I assume in this first example that there are four to eight participants, normally at Year 5 undergraduate or post-qualification level, and one facilitator.

A typical lesson plan would be as follows:

Stage 1:   Preparation and scene setting
(If necessary, give a reminder that 'We're here to help each other, not to criticise')

Here are the Student Notes for this scenario. When you've read them, we'll begin . . . and a word of advice – whatever happens, don't lose your temper!

5–10 minutes

Stage 2: Role play
Role play runs without interruption, with a single student taking the part of the doctor

8–15 minutes

Stage 3: Feedback
Many communication specialists ask for feedback following 'Pendleton's Rules.' That is, the person playing the doctor talks about 'What went well', and then the others join in on the same topic. Then the person playing the doctor talks about 'What might have been handled differently', and the others follow suit. This is occasionally helpful (qualified doctors might feel more vulnerable than students, who have less professional respect to lose) but usually, I think, imposes an artificial shape on a conversation where trust ought to be deeply embedded rather than supported by an overt structure.

The general shape of feedback is often as follows:

1 From role-playing doctor – a need to relax and offload ('Dear me [or possibly a bit stronger], that was hard . . . I completely lost it when . . . I had no idea what to say when he asked me if . . .).

2 Appropriate reassurance from audience.

3 General discussion – facilitator nudges discussion first on to details of the participant's communication, but notes other issues arising:
'Yes, the way he managed to persuade Mr Stafford to sit down was excellent – what was it he did, precisely, that made it happen?'

'I agree, we need to think in terms of rebuilding the relationship – let's come back to the concept of "relationships at work" later.'

4 Summary of key strengths and weaknesses of the participant's communication, usually delivered by facilitator.

5 Other matters arising – dealing with conflict, explaining risk and uncertainty, building professional relationships, etc.

15–40 minutes

Stage 4: Round-up

2–5 minutes

This gives a session of between 30 and 70 minutes, depending on how much time is available.

I've set out the scenario as consisting of participant notes, role player's notes and scenario notes.

Participant notes

(*See* above.) This is the information which the students receive before they meet the role player. They are asked to read it and to reflect on it. Given that in this case the student who is to play the part of the doctor is being asked to imagine a previous meeting with the patient's wife and son, it is worth spending a few seconds bringing that to life for them, and also saying 'You can assume that at the previous meeting you did nothing that you need to worry about.'

Role player's notes

This, obviously, is the brief that the role player is given several days in advance. Note a basic point of sensible practice – the possible age range for the role player is between about 25 and 45 years, and the scenario can be played by either a man or a woman (with the previous meeting with the GP involving the patient's partner). This is the version for a male role player. As a general rule, the wider the range of individuals who can play a scenario, the easier it is to find someone available to do it.

The role-player notes are extensive. It is absolutely central to this kind of enterprise that the character that is being presented is three-dimensional. To write a scenario in which, say, the only thing that matters is that the role player is hard of hearing is to reduce a person to a set of symptoms as surely as doctors are sometimes accused of doing. To give the character depth also enriches the discussion.

Scenario notes

These are notes for the participants to take away, serving as a reminder to them of what has taken place. It will be obvious that, in a context where one is not able to control with certainty the direction of discussion (any scenario has an infinite range of possibilities), one cannot guarantee that all and only the things which are mentioned here will be covered. However, I don't believe that this matters very much.

Role player's notes

You are Mr Oliver Stafford, a primary school teacher. You are married to Hilary, also a teacher, and have one son, Thomas, aged 5. Your wife took Thomas to see the GP a week ago with stomach pains, diarrhoea and loss of appetite. The GP examined Thomas and told your wife that he probably had a viral illness and that he should rest at home and take plenty of fluids but no food for 24 hours. She was also advised to contact the GP, or the deputising service out of hours, if his condition worsened.

Later that evening, while you were looking after Thomas alone (your wife was at a PTA meeting), he complained that the pains had got worse and moved over to the right-hand side of his stomach. You phoned and attended another GP at the out-of-hours service, who immediately made a provisional diagnosis of appendicitis. She was a little surprised that it hadn't been picked up earlier, and she sent Thomas straight to the hospital. He was examined by the surgeon on call, who confirmed that it was appendicitis. However, because you had given Thomas a drink of chocolate milk before leaving for the out-of-hours GP service, the anaesthetist refused to perform the operation for several (3–4) hours. At operation, Thomas was found to have an acutely inflamed appendix which, according to the surgeon, 'showed signs of perforation.' The surgeon also told you that the diagnosis was 'obvious', and that they were surprised that the GP had 'missed' it.

You have come to the GP today to demand an explanation for the misdiagnosis and to find out whether they were negligent or not. You still feel guilty about giving Thomas a drink and delaying his operation, but you were only carrying out the GP's instructions as relayed by your wife. You are not happy that you couldn't get through to the deputising service (shouldn't another line be installed for emergencies?), and you are unlikely to leave this consultation completely reassured. Whether you pursue the matter further will depend on how you are handled. Is the GP apologetic? Does the apology mask underlying negligence? Should you get a second opinion? Surely it is very easy to diagnose appendicitis? Does the explanation sound plausible? Don't leave until all your questions have been satisfactorily answered.

An undisclosed agenda is the tension between you and your wife. You are less successful than her in your work, and you very much want to be seen as a good father who has done the right thing.

Thomas is now making a good recovery at home.

Scenario notes

These notes are divided into:
1 a brief statement of aims
2 a set of bullet points listing the things that the 'good doctor' would do, which should provide you with the essential take-home messages for consultations of this kind
3 a 'background' section designed to examine the issues in more depth, and to

offer you a starting point for deeper reflection should you wish to pursue the issues now or in the future.

Note that this scenario relies on you 'remembering' a previous fictitious meeting with Mrs Stafford and her son – the rule of the game here is that you may assume you did nothing wrong during that consultation.

On the face of it, this scenario exists simply to provide an opportunity for you to practise and reflect on ways of handling aggression. This is obviously central to a successful consultation, but in fact there are a great many more things that you need to consider and reflect on.

1 The good doctor's aims for this consultation would be . . .

Well, clearly they would be defined and refined as you go along, because you don't know why Mr Stafford is here at the outset. However, fundamentally the aims are as follows:

- Improve your relationship with Mr Stafford, and by extension with the rest of the family, by:
  - demonstrating understanding and concern
  - helping Mr Stafford to understand why you acted as you did.

2 The good doctor would . . .

- Avoid confrontation/argument as far as possible (don't lose your temper).
- Listen patiently to Mr Stafford's initial narrative. You need to know what his starting point is. Expect him to do most of the talking early on.
- Ask after Thomas at an early stage. *So where is Thomas now? Is he at home? Is he recovering OK?* An offer to visit him is sometimes well received.
- Reassure Mr Stafford that he did the right thing in taking Thomas to Accident and Emergency. *You did exactly the right thing . . .*
- As soon as possible, show that you understand how much distress Thomas's illness must have caused. *That must have been very frightening for you . . .*
- Avoid the phrase *I understand how you feel*, or the equivalent. This is a gift (*Oh no you don't!*) for an angry patient.
- Clearly distinguish between your concern about shortcomings in the service that you provide (the problem with the deputising service needs to be looked into) and your concern that the Staffords have endured a very stressful few days. If you say *I'm sorry* (most people do in this scenario), be clear whether this is an admission of responsibility or not. Distinguish between *I'm sorry that this has happened* and *I'm sorry that I did the wrong thing.*
- If you make any promises, keep them. If you say *I'll look into this business of the deputising service and let you know*, make sure that you do.

- When Mr Stafford is sufficiently calm to take in what you say, explain clearly and succinctly why you didn't refer Thomas when you saw him.
- Don't get drawn into criticism of a fellow professional. *Well, I don't want to comment on what the consultant said.*
- Mr Stafford will almost certainly ask about the complaints procedure at the practice. Explain this calmly, and make it easy for him to see the Practice Manager.
- If things go well, confirm to Mr Stafford that it was appropriate for him to share his upset. *This has obviously been a difficult meeting for us both, but I'm glad you came in today.*
- Make sure that you yourself are calm and able to concentrate before you invite your next patient in – this is often known as 'housekeeping.'[a]

3 Background

BUILDING RELATIONSHIPS

This kind of scenario is often used in communication skills courses, not just in the health professions but also in other walks of life, and it is usually dealt with under the general heading of 'Difficult patients' or 'Dealing with aggression.' However, the problem with which Mr Stafford confronts the doctor is more complicated than that, and while one of your aims as you undertake, observe or reflect on the scenario must of course be to develop strategies for dealing with aggression, there are other issues as well.

Most people are aware that patients come to the doctor with problems which have clinical, social and psychological dimensions. This is known as the 'Triaxial Consultation', and it dates back to a Royal College of General Practitioners Working Paper published in 1972.

However, there are two other relevant dimensions which are always present to a greater or lesser extent, namely the *ethical* dimension and the *interpersonal* dimension. With most 'difficult patients', the issue of the interpersonal relationship is likely to be prominent. However, bear in mind one of the most basic but also most relevant of all insights into language – every time you have a conversation you express ideas, and at the same time you build, change, reconfirm and develop the relationship that you have with the other speaker(s).[b]

A golden rule – in the more discursive specialties, and those where a relationship continues over a long period of time (general practice and psychiatry are obvious examples), if you don't have an appropriate professional relationship with your patient, you will be able to achieve much less. For this reason, the most important aim for you today is to restore something of your relationship with the Staffords.

DEALING WITH AGGRESSION

This is obviously – at least at the start – a dysfunctional consultation, and one with the potential to get worse rather than better. Here is a typical opening:

> *Doctor:* Mr Stafford? What can I do –
>
> *Mr S:* What you can do for me is tell me why your bloody incompetence nearly cost my child his life –
>
> *Doctor:* Would you like to sit down?
>
> *Mr S:* No thanks. I'll stand . . .

. . . and so on. Mr Stafford's basic tactic, in other words, is not to play by the rules of the game – not to begin by sitting down and telling the doctor his problem, but to stand while the doctor tells *him* something. The doctor's task, in one sense, is quite simply to fashion an ordered consultation from this subversive beginning.

Typically, if the consultation is handled well, it will run something like this:

- Stage 1. Long tirade from Mr Stafford, as he unburdens himself of his anger and anxiety, and gives his narrative.
- Stage 2. Clarification of matters of fact by the doctor, before or as part of Stage 3.
- Stage 3. Explanation of previous course of action by doctor.
- Stage 4. Negotiation of the way forward.

Note therefore that if the consultation is successful it will in fact tend to have the overall shape and characteristics of what seems to have been the classic GP consultation for generations.[c] In other words, Mr Stafford will begin by doing most of the talking, with the doctor beginning to do more as an explanation is offered, and with both parties negotiating together towards the end.

Above all, therefore, let Mr Stafford have his say – don't interrupt unless you absolutely have to. In the end, he *will* stop, and if he is not confronted he will be less angry as a result. The other advantage of saying nothing is that it allows you to listen to Mr Stafford's version of the problem, in his own words. This is at the heart of the contemporary fashion for narrative-based medicine,[d] which has its antecedents in the famous dictum from around 1904, attributed to Sir William Osler and quoted in slightly different forms – 'Listen to the patient: he is telling you the diagnosis.'

This is a scenario which is, at one level, about dealing with anger, and therefore about conflict resolution.

The literature on anger and aggression is vast, and covers everything from the origins of warfare to assertiveness training.

Within primary care, you may find Naish *et al.*[e] helpful, although their message is to a large extent that 'Negative management tactics such as patient appeasement and exclusion are the norm.' They advocate involving the whole team in workshops, etc. to develop ways of coping.

With regard to strategies for defusing anger in the kind of one-to-one situation described here, most of what is available is (like the bullet points above) essentially anecdotal and common sense. It ranges from basic advice (don't raise your voice, try to encourage the other person to sit down if they are refusing to do so), to protecting yourself (place yourself between the angry patient and the door, or – potentially contradictory advice – stay within range of your panic button, if you have one), to discussion of formal models.

Among studies of conflict in the workplace, the best known is that by Thomas and Kilmann.[f] They suggest two dimensions, namely assertiveness and cooperation, as shown in Figure 4.1.

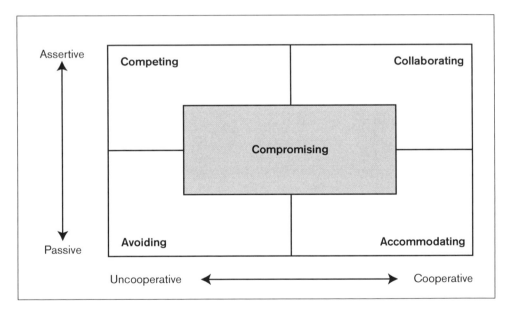

FIGURE 4.1

Each individual has their own preferred style for handling conflict, and any particular conflict can be imagined as lying somewhere on the graph in Figure 4.1.

The authors emphasise that no one style is always better than another, although in fact it is clear enough that a 'collaborating' style, in which the objectives of both participants are met at a 'high' level, is actually to be considered the ideal.

You can take a questionnaire on-line (and free) from which your own preferred style can be derived. To some people this kind of model (hundreds of which are used on professional training courses) seems brilliantly to encapsulate a key issue, whereas to others it seems slick and shallow. At any rate, the original instrument, although over 30 years old, is still used, often as a jumping-off point for looking at cross-cultural negotiation[g] – some cultures are said to 'avoid', some 'compete', and so on. However, such labels must be used with care! They can very easily slip over into stereotypical nonsense.

The key point to bear in mind, and the thing you need to understand as you talk to Mr Stafford, is that this kind of aggression is symptomatic – in this case of anxiety and fear. If there is a single maxim to learn from this scenario it is that angry people are seldom wicked.

However, 'managing aggression' is not an end in itself, nor can it be achieved in a context-free manner. In cases of political conflict, one must remove the immediate heat from a situation (make the players less angry) *because* this is a prerequisite for helping all involved to comprehend the logic of each other's position, *because* this in turn is a prerequisite for rebuilding trust, *because* this – finally – is the basis on which the next steps can be taken and the nature of the future relationship between the parties consolidated. The case in this scenario is no different. Defusing the immediate anger is the first step, but there are many further steps to be undertaken, not all of which will be possible at this meeting, no doubt, but the GP here should have the longer term in mind.

EXPLAINING UNCERTAINTY

One of the difficulties is that the logic of the GP's position is complex, and for an angry and distressed parent, too subtle for him easily to have patience with.

Usually, the doctor tries to explain that if all children who just *might* have appendicitis were sent off to hospital the system would grind to a halt. Interestingly, this part of the scenario is seldom handled particularly well, even by experienced GPs.

What we are considering here is how we talk about risk and uncertainty. This is an important generic issue, and one therefore which is well worth thinking through. (A recent study of doctors dealing with possible meningitis parallels the issues in this scenario very closely.[h]) Note that at least under certain circumstances,[i] and probably under most circumstances in primary care, doctors are more likely to express uncertainty about the clinical problem than the patient is, and the ability to remain uncertain while retaining the patient's trust is extremely important.

In many jobs there are instances of risk and uncertainty which are encountered repeatedly. Most people will develop a set way of saying something which seems to work for the patient, but which also works for the doctor (they feel the words represent the case truly, the words suit their own style of speech, etc.). Here is an anaesthetist, the day before an operation:

> I'm obliged to tell you there's a risk attached to all anaesthesia. But to be frank you probably ran a greater risk driving to the hospital this morning.

Perhaps that might work for you, or perhaps not. For Mr Stafford, perhaps:

> You'll know as a parent how often children get little tummy upsets and that kind of thing. And usually it's nothing. So what we have to do as doctors is to wait and see how things develop. The alternative is that people get worried and the hospital system gets overloaded.

This kind of explanation is better delivered slowly, if possible (this may be difficult if Mr Stafford is still – as he will have been at the start – eager to fill every space in the conversation with invective). Then, all being well, you can go on to an explanation of the importance of safety-netting,[a] and an acknowledgement that your safety-netting arrangements didn't work, apparently because of a problem with the deputising service.

This raises an important point. Although the scenario is set up so that the doctor may assume that the previous clinical examination and management of the problem were entirely appropriate, it appears clear that the practice must accept responsibility for Mr Stafford's inability to contact the deputising service.

Or at least this is probably so, which brings us to a consideration of evidence.

EVIDENCE

No, not clinical evidence, but the evidence of memory. Mr Stafford will probably tell the doctor something like this:

> *Mr S:* I was on the phone non-stop for about 45 minutes trying to get someone to pick up at the other end. I tried dozens of times – sometimes the phone just rang and rang, sometimes I got the engaged tone – in the end I gave up, because Thomas was in so much distress . . .

The question here is what you should believe. Perhaps Mr Stafford's account is strictly and precisely true, but I doubt it. Perhaps what he really means is that he tried once, the phone wasn't answered immediately, his son demanded his attention, he hung up, and this pattern repeated itself three or four times over a 20-minute period. Maybe that's actually the truth of the matter. No angry person ever underestimates the grounds for their anger when talking to the person whom they see as the guilty party.

Nevertheless, it sounds as if something is not working as it should do. Memory allows us, if we are not very careful, to persuade ourselves that our case is stronger than we think, and that things really did happen the way we remember them. And bear in mind also that Mr and Mrs Stafford have had opportunities since the crisis to reinforce their own view of events.

In other words, there is too much hearsay drifting about your meeting with Mr Stafford for much of it to be absolutely reliable. Weighing the evidence is part of good listening, too.

NOISES OFF

The main question here is why Mr Stafford has come today, when it was Mrs Stafford who was at the original meeting. And the answer is, probably, that you'll never know. Perhaps, earlier at home, Mr Stafford has said something like *'Right, you leave this to me. I know what you're like, you'll just give in to him . . .'.* Patients bring only a small part of their lives into the surgery.

Note that it is built into the role player's brief here that Mrs Stafford has a more successful career than her husband. Therefore underpinning some of the distress that Mr Stafford brings to the surgery is (to a greater or lesser extent) is his desire to reassert his authority in the home.

Reflection

This is a role play, not reality, and the scenario is deliberately set up so that you may assume your conduct during the previous consultation with Mrs Stafford and Thomas was fine. Yet a fair number of students over the years report feelings of guilt when they talk to Mr Stafford, a sense of anxiety that after all the criticism might be justified.

In a climate in which patients are more willing to complain, any doctor is likely to face unjustified criticism. It's worth thinking now, in advance, about how you would try to cope with this.

Suggested reading

a Neighbour R. *The Inner Consultation.* 2nd ed. Oxford: Radcliffe Publishing; 2004. For many people, still the single most important text on medical communication. It aims to be inspirational, and everyone should at least be familiar with its main points.

b Halliday MAK. *Explorations in the Function of Language.* London: Edward Arnold; 1973. You need a very serious interest in language to read this (so don't, unless you really, really want to grapple with something difficult), but Halliday's basic distinction, echoed here, has been very influential.

c Byrne P, Long B. *Doctors Talking to Patients.* London: HMSO; 1976. A classic in its day, and one of the starting points for modern medical communication studies. Curiously, it is still sometimes quoted as if it was contemporary in all respects.

d Greenhalgh T, Hurwitz B. *Narrative-Based Medicine.* London: BMJ Books; 1998. An interesting and insightful approach.

e Naish J, Carter YH, Gray RW *et al.* Brief encounters of aggression and violence in primary care: a team approach to coping strategies. *Fam Pract.* 2002; **19:** 504–10.

f Thomas KW, Kilmann RH. *Thomas–Kilmann Conflict Mode Instrument.* Mountain View, CA: Xicom Incorporated; 1974.

g Samarah I, Paul S, Mykytyn P. Exploring the links between cultural diversity, the collaborative conflict management style, and performance of global virtual teams. In: Banker RD, Chang H, Kao Y-C, editors. *Proceedings of the Eighth Americas Conference on Information Systems.* Atlanta, GA: Association for Information Systems; 2002.

h Brennan CA, Somerset M, Granier SK *et al.* Management of diagnostic uncertainty in children with possible meningitis: a qualitative study. *Br J Gen Pract.* 2003; **53:** 626–31.

i Skelton JR, Murray J, Hobbs FDR. Imprecision in medical communication: study of a doctor talking to patients with serious illness. *J R Soc Med.* 1999: **92:** 620–5.

References

1 James H. Preface to The author of Beltraffio. In: *The Art of the Novel.* New York: Charles Scribner's Sons; 1934. p. 236.

2 Smith SR, Cookson J, Mckendree J *et al.* Patient-centred learning: back to the future. *Med Teacher.* 2007; **29:** 33–7.

CHAPTER 5

The rules of the game

As an unperfect actor on the stage
Who with his fear is put besides his part . . .

(William Shakespeare, Sonnet 23[1])

Introduction

The point about conflicts is that they are, by definition, dysfunctional situations. Mr Stafford cannot be assisted until a functional relationship exists, and in general a conflict cannot be resolved until the relationship has been repaired. Yet although the literature on the 'health professional–patient' relationship is vast, it tends not to deal with such questions as how one repairs relationships, nor with the need to understand and play by the rules of the game.

I shall now turn to the cases of two individuals who either do not know how to or do not choose to follow the rules. As you read, you might like to consider the extent to which the problems raised here are problems which are best thought of as communication issues, or as something else. In the case of Gerry Parker, who is the first person we meet, you might or might not like to think of this as a clinical issue (the advice to the role player, however, is not to handle the role in such a way as to make a clinical approach obviously appropriate). In the second case, you might like to reflect on the extent to which the GP might be portrayed as unethical, or as briefly in a panic – and whether being in a panic is an appropriate defence against the accusation of unethical conduct. However, in both cases the ordinary battery of communication skills strategies takes one only so far.

Both of these scenarios are appropriate at undergraduate level. Post-qualification, participants find the issues easier to resolve, and seldom become entangled in the kind of polite refusals that – as we shall see – can be very problematical.

We shall assume lesson plans with a similar overall shape to that presented in the previous chapter. An alternative range of possibilities, for larger groups, is outlined in Chapter 7.

Rich context scenario 2: The case of the lonely designer

(Note that this is a scenario that was briefly mentioned in *Language and Clinical Communication*).

Participant notes

You are a GP in surgery. Your next patient is Geraldine Parker. You see from the notes that she has recently registered, having moved up from London. This is your first consultation with her.

Role player's notes

You are Geraldine ('Call me Gerry . . .') Parker, a graphic designer from London who has just moved to another big city as a design consultant for a major department store. You know no one locally, you live in a flat on your own and you are quite lonely. When you were a student in London you met and dated a number of medical students and, briefly, a couple of doctors. You have always found medics good fun to be with. In the past, you have reacted badly to isolation and living on your own, and at one stage you had a 'breakdown' of sorts (at least that is the label you use privately to yourself when you think about that period of your life), and became temporarily dependent on temazepam (a sleeping tablet).

■ If the participant is male, you are looking for a date.
■ If the participant is female, you're looking for a 'best girlfriend' for going out – there are no lesbian overtones, and you should clearly signal that you are straight if asked.

You have heard that one of the doctors in your local practice is very nice, and you decide to use a consultation to meet him or her. Your initial pretence is that you want some general health advice (diet, exercise, contraception, etc., *but don't get hung up on any of them – the point is that you want to make contact with the doctor*). You are quite happy to talk about your past sexual history. If the doctor appears uninterested, you could mention your previous problem with sleeping tablets. Try to manipulate the consultation so that the subject comes round to personal questions about the doctor's home/social life – 'What do you like doing in the evenings?', 'Can we meet for a drink?', 'You must have a girlfriend – haven't you!?', 'By the way, that colour really suits you', 'I can sense we've got a lot in common', 'Where can you have a nice intimate drink round here?', and so on.

If you hit a brick wall at every turn, ask the student if they would go out with you if you weren't a patient. Then offer to switch doctors and suggest that you cook a meal for them. You might perhaps even ask to be examined.

Scenario notes

So what did you make of this woman?

The good doctor's aims
- Develop a relationship of trust with the patient.
- Leave her in no doubt that the relationship between doctor and patient must be therapeutic.

The good doctor would . . .
- Take the patient seriously, aware that her perhaps strange presentation of herself deserves sympathy and understanding.
- Remain courteous at all times.
- Quickly recognise that the patient had no clear conception of the doctor–patient relationship.
- Quickly realise that the patient had difficulty in recognising polite refusals.
- Be aware of the possibility of clinical issues, but probably decide not to explore them at this stage, because the overriding requirement would be for the doctor to make clear to the patient that they were trustworthy, and could offer assistance with problems which would appropriately be addressed to a doctor.

Background

This scenario, to be frank, was originally created as a little light relief for the role players and participants alike. We envisaged an opportunity for the former to ham things up a bit, for the latter to try to avoid giggling and, if they struggled to cope, for them both to endure some (friendly, we would hope) teasing from colleagues. However, this is not how it turned out.

The scenario plays differently, on the whole, depending on whether the doctor is male or female. With a female doctor in particular the overall presentation can be embarrassing to observe, even a little creepy, and often very sad.

The point about this patient is that she doesn't play the game by the rules

– the game of 'doctors and patients' at one level, but the game of human interaction at another. This is built into the scenario, in words like 'pretence' and 'manipulate', which as you see are in the role player's notes. The point is that the patient's behaviour is inappropriate, and for that matter she is inappropriately persistent in her approach. Most of us have a moderately clear idea of the boundaries between our private self and the self we present to the world on public occasions, such as visiting a doctor and playing the role of patient, or playing the role of customer in a shop, or of parent at a school parents' evening, and so on. However, Gerry does not.

Sometimes the occasion is so unusual that the rules are made explicit. The rules of the very British game 'How to be presented to the Queen' appear to be something like this, for example:

> Do not speak until the Queen speaks to you.
> She will offer her hand and say 'How do you do?'
> Shake her hand, and say 'How do you do Your Majesty?'
> Do not say anything else unless the Queen speaks to you again.
> If she does, address her as 'Ma'am.'

However, most of the time we understand the rules as we go along – we understand what is appropriate in particular circumstances. (It isn't appropriate, when a policeman flags us down for driving too fast, to begin a discussion with him about where he went on holiday last year, and so on). And, if someone says something unwelcome to us, we know how to let them down politely ('I wish I could come – but I'm already going out that night . . .').

This is all part of the way in which language works. A major part of communication is concerned with matching my intention when I say something to your interpretation of what I say. If I can't offer appropriate clues, I have a problem – if you can't pick them up, you have a problem.

Gerry's problem is, at least on the surface, that she has little ability to pick up clues. The doctor's problem is to establish a proper therapeutic relationship.

This is one of the scenarios that we use where there is a very clear difference between the level of competence of a qualified doctor and that of a medical student – even one in their final year, which is when this scenario tends to be worked on. The real problem for the doctor is to find language of sufficient clarity to make their position clear, while not hurting Gerry's feelings and making her feel – no doubt for the hundredth time – that she has been rejected. Medical students find this very difficult.

So, for example, a common approach will be something like this (we'll assume the doctor is female):

D: Ms Parker?

P: Hi, call me Gerry – ooh, that's a lovely bracelet. [*Gerry sits down, and reaches out to touch the bracelet on the doctor's arm*]. Do you mind me asking – where did you get it?

D: Oh, in town somewhere, I'm not sure now –

P: Really? Everyone's been telling me the shopping is great here – I'm new to the area, don't have anyone to show me around really . . .

Thus, 10 seconds into the conversation, the doctor is on the point of receiving a suggestion that she and Gerry meet up and go shopping together ('You've obviously got my kind of taste – anyway, I was wanting to buy some clothes for this new job I'm starting, you know the people there aren't as friendly as I was hoping they would be . . .').

Almost always, the doctor will respond in line with a set of conventions that simply don't work. They will assume that Gerry has an ability to deal with the world which she simply lacks. So, in response to the shopping offer, they might say something like 'Well, I can't really, I don't seem to have much free time . . .'

This statement about availability is, functionally, a polite refusal, as we at once recognise. If someone said it to us, we would feel that we were being gently turned away, unless the speaker went out of their way to say otherwise – 'I really *don't* have any free time at present – but maybe in a couple of weeks . . .?'

Gerry's problem is that she simply doesn't recognise a refusal when she hears one. A typical reply will therefore be something along the lines of 'They must give you some time, surely? Saturday night – how about that? We could go for a meal . . .'

Gerry is relentless, and until the doctor feels able to stop making polite excuses, the embarrassment is prolonged. With a male participant, the point will come when Gerry mentions that she used to go out with a doctor – 'I've always liked doctors for some reason. Maybe it's because they're always so caring, and they know so much . . . You remind me of a doctor I used to see quite a lot of, actually . . .' Something this blatant will help the doctor to dig in his heels, but even here the terms of the refusal are often insufficiently robust, because they are too polite:

P: Maybe we could go out for a meal – you know, just for a chat . . .

D: No, I couldn't do that, I'm afraid – it's not ethical to have that sort of relationship with a patient.

> P: Oh, I wasn't suggesting anything . . . Anyway, how would it be if I registered with another doctor, then we could meet . . .

By this time the doctor is certainly thinking 'There are absolutely no circumstances under which I would like you to be my girlfriend' – which, sadly, is what men usually think about Gerry, one can tell.

So, in the end, the doctor has to step back from the interaction, and address the issue completely straightforwardly: 'My relationship with you is therapeutic. I would like to work with you as your doctor. I'm happy to support you with any health problems you have or may have in the future. But I'm not happy to enter into any other kind of relationship.'

The central moral of this scenario is that unless the relationship is appropriate, it cannot easily be of therapeutic value. Clearly this is particularly true here, because of the nature of Gerry's 'health problem', and we shall turn to that now.

You will see from the role player's brief that Gerry has previously been on antidepressants, and this is intended to signal to the role player that there is some kind of pervasive unhappiness in Gerry's life. It is up to the role player how evident this is, provided always that her surface presentation is apparently bright and cheerful. Almost always she will give hints of some profound distress, but there will never be a well-defined cause of this. This means that it will be clear that the bare minimum aim for this consultation is to keep the channel open – not to send Gerry away feeling that she can't come back again, and not to send her away thinking that, in general, 'doctors don't want to know.' You will inescapably have the feeling that this is someone who is going to need your professional services. And in fact, from time to time, the discussion after the role play can centre on whether it's worth assessing her mental health immediately.

However, it is harder to tell how and why to intervene in this case, so she raises issues of what we mean when we say someone is 'ill', and what we mean when we say that, as doctors, our time is well spent. Would we not be better off spending our time with that patient over there, who has a well-defined condition which we happen to know will respond well to intervention? Or, alternatively, by putting the effort into supporting Gerry now, and perhaps seeing her regularly over a period of time (usually for nothing much), might we prevent some disaster – a suicide, perhaps?

And as a result of both of these things, Gerry invites discussion about the handling of uncertainty. She is a profoundly ambiguous character, and invites anyone who meets her to think about how comfortable they are with this level of ambiguity. If you enjoy the challenge of meeting her, and take pleasure in resolving the immediate situation so that the beginnings of a therapeutic relationship exist, then perhaps a career choice like general practice is for you. And if not, perhaps it is not.

Ideas for reflection

This is a meeting which begins dysfunctionally and runs the risk of remaining dysfunctional. There are probably two levels at which it is worth reflecting on this. One is within the context of what we know of 'doctor–patient relationships', although this tends to concentrate on the extent to which doctors and patients should have a 'mutualistic' relationship or (a way of looking at it which remains popular within medical education) an 'adult–adult' relationship, in the sense in which such labels are used by transactional analysts. The other approach is to consider it in terms of the rules of ordinary social interaction.

There is of course a third way, namely to consider what Gerry says, and the way she presents more generally, as evidence of a clinical problem – but the role player's presentation usually avoids that.

The other question is whether or not Gerry has either a clinical problem (and therefore a right to your attention) or a problem with life (and if so what right she has to your attention, if any).

THE DOCTOR–PATIENT RELATIONSHIP

1 What different types of doctor–patient relationship have been proposed? What do you understand by them? Is one type better than another?

Here is one well-known breakdown:

Patient control	Doctor control	
	Low	High
Low	Default	Paternalism
High	Consumerism	Mutuality

(*see* Stewart and Roter 1989,[a] p. 21)

2 Do you think that continuity of care (or having a 'personal doctor') matters? How far should the doctor keep their private self and their public self apart?

Here is an extract from an interview with a GP in a rural practice. He is thinking about the relationship between the private and the personal, and about the extent to which patients know about him as a person, as well as the extent to which he knows about their lives. As you read, ask yourself the following questions.

■ Is this what I personally think medicine is 'about'? (Is this mix of the <u>private</u> and the <u>public</u> what, ultimately, we mean by 'holistic care'?)

- Could I be described as an 'open' person? If so, what does this suggest about my career choices? (Do you need to be 'open' to be a GP?)
- Is the time that the doctor quoted below probably spends on social chat appropriate or not?

D: But . . . it is marvellous I I I I work in a rural mixed [inaudible] practice and . . . there it's very much y'know the GP . . . who I take make decisions and . . . people don't really want necessarily to consider options they want me to decide.

I: Yeah yeah.

D: Which in many ways is old-fashioned . . . the usefulness of continuity [as a] GP to get to know the person so you have that intimate knowledge of their I was saying this to somebody . . . on the way down it's just extraordinary that intimate knowledge we have of people's lives and that that's very useful to that's a very useful means of continuing to sort of generate this mutual trust you have.

I: Yeah.

D: This sort of openness about my own life and their lives so that there's a y'know what I'm doing in my life that forms part of the consultation.

I: Yes.

D: I don't have a problem with that personally and I I'm by nature an open person anyway.

I: OK . . .

D: . . . But I think I find y'know sometimes life as a GP is difficult when I feel like I'm trying I'm taking over I have too much responsibility in regard to this person.

I: Yes.

D: Or too much is expected of me maybe relatives or family and I then personally feel I'm taking on too much responsibility.

I: Yeah.

D: Which is stressful.

I: Yes.

D: And y'know maybe something I have to teach myself it's not not to take on too much responsibility for other people's lives and . . . in the matter in the matter of y'know [inaudible] end-of-life decisions this sort of thing [I'm] inclined perhaps

to to take to take all too much responsibility and of course the key as somebody else said in y'know in day-to-day life 'Are you ready for the next patient?' . . .
(Data courtesy of Irish College of General Practice, and Dr M O'Riordan)

Look at the literature on this.[b–e]

PLAYING BY THE RULES

Gerry seems not to know how to conduct normal relationships. She doesn't know the rules of the interactional game. These rules are intricate, heavily nuanced and context dependent. Yet we expect everyone, including ourselves, to know them. Consider some basic rules – for example, what is the range of things you can say when the phone rings and you pick it up?

Well, you can give your number, or your name, or say 'Hello', or 'Good morning' . . . and not too much else. However, you can't (as Spaniards can) lift up the phone and say 'Speak to me' (*'Digame'*).

Can you think of other situations which are rule governed in this way?

We avoid rudeness by being indirect. We don't say 'You look awful in that tight shirt', but 'I always think you look better in something more free-flowing . . .'

Gerry's problem is that she can't take a hint. You will almost certainly see her being offered a series of polite refusals to her requests that she doesn't notice. This means – and it's a skill needed by teachers as well as by health professionals – that you need to be able to speak very directly to her. Most students find this difficult.

RATIONING

One of the issues with Gerry is the extent to which she is using the healthcare services appropriately. Do you think that she is doing so? Is this a question of 'rationing'?

Here is an extract from a much cited paper published in 1997:[f]

> When the argument that 'rationing is inevitable' is applied not to situations with effectively absolute shortages like liver transplants, but to the healthcare system as a whole, it assumes that there can never be enough money, or surgeons or drugs or child psychiatrists, to satisfy all the needs that people have. Interestingly, I hear this argument most in Britain, which spends the least money from direct taxes trying to meet those needs and demands. And I don't hear it from ordinary citizens, only from people with university degrees. Ordinary citizens tell me about a family member who is not getting adequate care for a serious health problem and wonder why. They don't know that they could get it if they were in a nation

with an adequately funded free health service with no waiting lists, like Holland or Germany.

Do you agree? Or, to put it another way, would the demands that Gerry might make on the practice be (a) 'infinite' or (b) more than the practice could cope with? (Or, an entirely different question, would bringing Gerry into the healthcare system merely encourage her to somatise life's problems, and so add to the health service burden of caring for illness the burden of caring for manufactured illness?)

A final word on the doctor–patient relationship. A genuine partnership between a doctor and a patient involves more than words. Any doctor can say 'I think we should do X. What do you think?' Any doctor can elicit a response ('That's fine'), which might or might not come from the heart. However, a genuine partnership depends not just on the words of the moment, but on the underlying relationship – which takes us back both to the need to offer Gerry something genuine, and which she understands, and to the fact that it doesn't matter so much what you say, as whether the relationship in which it is contextualised is appropriate, and healthy.

Suggested reading

a Stewart M, Roter D. Introduction. In: Stewart M, Roter D, editors. *Communicating with Medical Patients*. Newbury Park, CA: Sage; 1989. p. 21.

b Di Blasi Z, Harkness E, Ernst E *et al*. Influence of context effects on health outcomes: a systematic review. *Lancet*. 2001; **357**: 757–62.

c Howie JGR, Heaney DJ, Maxwell M *et al*. Quality at general practice consultations: cross-sectional survey. *BMJ*. 1999; **319**: 738–43.

d Ettlinger P, Freeman G. General practice compliance study: is it worth being a personal doctor? *BMJ*. 1981; **282**: 1192–4.

e Hjortdahl P, Laerum E. Continuity of care in general practice: effect on patient satisfaction. *BMJ*. 1992; **304**: 1287–90.

f Light DW. The real ethics of rationing. *BMJ*. 1997; **315**: 112–15.

Comment

The scenario notes here pre-empt much of what should be said by way of comment. However, it's important to add just one thing. Gerry's presentation is ambivalent – different role players tackle the role in different ways, some more over the top than others, some more evidently strange than others, but the end point is almost always a recognition by the participants that she is distressed. Whether this distress would benefit from a clinical label or not is an interesting discussion, but is not often central to the scenario, and on occasion

– precisely because the role player's task here is to push the participant to the point where there is no option but a straight and absolute refusal – the level of embarrassment can be genuinely difficult to watch.

At times, too, one thinks 'No, it would never get this far, even Gerry would get the message by this time and stop pushing.' This may be true, although we would all say that we have met people who 'couldn't take a hint' – but the point to stress is that role play is not necessarily realistic. It's a common misappprehension that it is, or that it ought to be. The actor's central goal may be to create a sense of belief (or, in the famous phrase, 'suspended disbelief') – the point of other kinds of simulation in the health professions (e.g. the use of mannikins) may be to make them as similar as possible to the real thing. However, the core of the role player's task is the creation of educational opportunity, not of a realistic illusion.

Here is another example of someone who cannot play the game – or at any rate, who tries not to. This is a scenario which raises serious ethical issues.

Rich context scenario 3: Alcohol and insight – on not being nice
Participant notes
You are the newest practice nurse recruited to a local GP surgery with five partners. You have been in the post for a month, and enjoy the work. You have not got to know the other staff socially yet, but they seem nice and are helpful. The other practice nurse, Rose Muller, has asked for a quick chat in your room. You have no indication what she wants to talk about.

Role player's notes
You are Rose Muller, one of two practice nurses in a five-partner practice in a small town. You have been working at the health centre for 8 years. The other nurse is new, having joined last month.

You used to genuinely love your job, and you always seemed to attract the patients with a lot of personal problems, many of whom would ask for you by name. This would mean that your consultations would last longer than the allocated time (10 minutes or so) and your clinics always ran late. You would therefore stay late and see extra patients in your lunch break.

Recently you have been overwhelmed by your workload, and you have been struggling to keep up. When patients come in with their seemingly endless 'moans', you feel disinclined to listen, and you feel that 'there just isn't enough of you to go round.' You recognise that this is a change, and the dismay you feel at the prospect of seeing another patient with a personal problem is very different from how you used to feel. Previously your job was a pleasure, and you always had a smile on your face as you walked through the door. Now you have started to dread going to work.

Socially, your family seem to be always nagging you because you are 'no fun any more' and you seem disengaged when you do visit them. You have lived alone for several years, and you don't have a partner to whom you can turn for advice and comfort. You have a small number of old friends, but have been declining more invitations than you accept of late, using a variety of plausible excuses – double bookings, minor colds and evening meetings.

In yourself you feel very low generally, and are experiencing difficulty sleeping at night. This has been going on for several months. There was no specific trauma or negative life event that precipitated it, just a creeping feeling of sadness and low mood. In addition, you find that you are somewhat weepy, and this can catch you out at almost any time.

The only thing that seems to help is alcohol, so you have been drinking more recently – in fact, the thought of the 'escape' of 'a few drinks' in the evening gets you through the day. On a typical night you might easily finish two bottles of wine, or occasionally more. However, you would not in any way perceive yourself as an alcoholic, 'because you only drink after work, not during the day.'

The main and more immediate problem today is that you have just been caught by the police for drink-driving and you have been warned that (a) the case will go to court and (b) you will probably lose your licence. It was a stupid mistake to make. You ran out of wine and drove a couple of miles to a local outlet for more.

You are going to have a chat with the new nurse at the practice. There are two problems:

1 You live in a village with poor transport links. If you lose your licence, getting to and from work will be a real concern. You've heard that the new nurse lives about 5 miles from you. Also, you work split-site (1.5 days at another surgery). This means that on a Friday you literally dash from one surgery to another, during a 30-minute window. There wouldn't be enough time to catch a bus, and taxis would be costly.

2 While the district nurses cover most of the home visits in the area, you do have one responsibility that the district team don't cover. This is with regard to influenza awareness, and involves visiting care homes in advance of winter. You see this as very worthwhile (and good for your CV). This activity would be a real headache without a car.

Perhaps if you can persuade your new colleague to help (cover for) you, you could come up with a plan together to keep things running smoothly without other staff finding out about your misdemeanour. There are several important points.

- You do <u>not</u> want the other staff in the practice to know about this (although this would contradict Royal College of Nursing guidelines).
- If you are asked, you admit to feeling depressed, but surely all clinical staff get a bit low sometimes?
- You don't want to admit that you may not be up to your job at present – you are sure that you will feel better soon.
- The alcohol is becoming a bit of a problem, but then all health professionals (especially the doctors) drink a lot, don't they?
- You don't want people to perceive you as a non-coper just because you have got 'a bit low.'

Comments

The problem with most students, then, is that they are fundamentally nice, and that consequently they don't play the game of being a health professional correctly. Part of this problem, it must be said, is the false dichotomy that gets set up in a great deal of clinical training – between the nice, approachable, empathic, holistic practitioner (hooray!) on the one hand, and the unpleasant, distant, unempathic, mechanistic individual (boo!) on the other. This can quickly be reduced to a view that, when it comes to communication, niceness is all. In fact, the situation is a lot more complex.

One of the overriding aims of most speakers is to preserve face – their own and other people's. So we don't say to our colleague 'No, you can't deal with that problem because you'd make a complete mess of it.' We say 'It might be better if Abdul does that – he's got more experience in that area than you have.' And if we are reasonably sensitive individuals we probably go away and work out for ourselves that we weren't considered to be completely competent, but were let down kindly. However, this only works when both parties know the game, as meeting Gerry Parker shows us. Both parties must have insight, and the ability to interpret a polite rebuff both as a rebuff (they know where they stand) and as polite (they don't take offence). It also means that both parties are well intentioned.

In other words, this scenario forces students to break the rules, just as Gerry Parker did. However, the situation here is worse, in the sense that we will witness a senior colleague deploying good communication skills ('good' in the sense that many famously nasty people have, sadly, been good communicators) in order to try to manipulate a more junior colleague.

And 'manipulative' is the keyword for the role player here. Their approach should be very task-focused – the aim is to get consent, by whatever means possible. This may involve some kind of surface signals of wheedling, but is more likely to be attempted through charm. In other words, the role player has to be someone it's hard to say 'no' to. And the best approach, from their point of view, may well be to attempt to get the student to buy into the deal at a very low level ('It'd be good for you to get out and about, see the patients in their own homes, get to know them a bit . . .'), so that there is a measure of acceptance given before the student realises quite what is being asked of them. This forces them into the more difficult position of having to backtrack from a promise that has already been half given.

No participant we have worked with has ever actually agreed to do what the health professional asks, so far as I am aware. This is encouraging, because it indicates that the ethical issue is clear even to relatively junior students, once the nurse comes sufficiently clean for them to understand what the deal actually is – they must enter into a kind of conspiracy with a colleague, and by extension help her to hide a problem which may have serious repercussions for patient care. It also means that they must find the words to make their position clear. In other words, 'I'd be scared to – what if I was found out?' isn't a suitable polite refusal, whereas 'No, Rose, I'm sorry – I'm afraid I think that wouldn't be the right thing to do' is.

It's worth noting the vast difference between inviting participants into this scenario without preparation, and inviting them to discuss the issues first. Using the latter approach means that everyone knows what they are supposed to do, and the only teaching point is the language of polite refusal, with everyone's attention consequently being very much on the surface behaviour of the two parties. Doing the scenario *without* preparation is an excellent way of finding out to what extent students have internalised the lessons of professionalism. Thinking one's way through ethical issues on the hoof, as it were, is not possible – students who have not previously reflected on what 'being professional' means will do badly. However, students who have understood the need to ask the question 'What is it to be a health professional?' will have a basis for responding appropriately to the inappropriate request.

This scenario, in other words, can be used at either a surface or a deep level (see *Language and Clinical Communication* for discussion of these terms), to address the issue either of the words that people use, or of the professionalism which you hope directs their use of words.

It is, of course, also a scenario which brings home to students the fact that communication isn't just something that happens with patients. The colleague-to-colleague context is potentially difficult, partly because it is under-taught, and partly because it is under-researched. A great deal of advice on colleague-to-colleague interaction comes from the business tradition, but this is often more a series of slogans than anything else, and while there are limits to what research can tell you in principle about how to communicate, there is the further difficulty with many of these books that they give an impression more of slickness (and, at worst, of self-publicising) than of profundity.

This is one of those scenarios which works rather badly at postgraduate level. Qualified professionals may sometimes still be bad at breaking bad news, say, but they don't often perform very poorly at saying this kind of difficult thing, or at understanding the need for clarity at the expense of accommodating the wishes of the other person if necessary. This is perhaps more to do with maturity and self-confidence than with anything else, and perhaps – to return to the Socratic model – it rests partly on the experienced professional's developing ability to help people to 'know themselves' better, in the famous phrase. This is the approach to the next scenario.

Reference

1   Shakespeare W. Sonnet 23. In: Jowett J, Montgomery W, Taylor G, Wells S, editors. *The Oxford Shakespeare: the complete works.* 2nd ed. Oxford: Oxford University Press; 2005. p. 781 (written *c.*1599–1609).

CHAPTER 6

Ask, don't tell

Every time we teach a child something, we keep him from inventing it by himself.

(Jean Piaget, *Some aspects of operations*[1])

Introduction

The Socratic lesson, it will be recalled, is to do with identifying one's ignorance or confusion as a result of being on the receiving end of persistent questions. In this chapter, we look at two individuals who need to be offered the opportunity to find out for themselves what their problems are. That is to say, in both cases what we are dealing with is an aspect of education – in the first case, the education of a patient, and in the second case, education under the aegis of appraisal.

As always with Socrates, the point is to elicit: to bring the other person to a state of articulating the problem, not of telling them what it is – however obvious that may be to you. And also, as we have seen, there is a tension in the Socratic lesson, in the western classroom – and as immediately below, in the consulting room – between encouraging and valuing the ideas of the other, and allowing them to get away with nonsense.

Scenario for elicitation 1: On not worrying

Participant notes

You are a GP in afternoon surgery. Your next patient is Cathleen Curtis. You have not seen her before. Her notes indicate that she attends four or five times a year, and there is no significant past medical history in her summary.

Role player's notes

You are Cathleen Curtis, an unmarried IT worker. You are in good physical health, although you have always been a bit of a worrier. Your mother died of breast cancer at the age of 55 years, and your father, aged 59 years, has recently had an operation to remove a cancer of the bowel, from which he is making a good recovery. You have had a bad psychological reaction to this and have become obsessed with the idea that you are going to develop cancer imminently.

You don't smoke, and you've only ever had one sexual partner (you've read that cervical cancer is related to sexual intercourse). You drink very occasionally and take care not to burn in the sun by wearing long sleeves and covering your legs in the summer, as well as avoiding foreign travel. You eat a healthy diet, swim twice a week, have regular smears (the last one, 6 months ago, was normal) and examine your breasts regularly. However, such is your phobia that you have recently taken to examining your breasts most days and keeping a mental note of your bowel habit (frequency, consistency and colour). You dislike eating any food unless you have prepared it yourself, and you have become 'paranoid' about passive smoking – so much so that you sometimes wear a surgical-style mask in very smoky environments, partly to 'make a point.' You don't like being too close to anyone in case you catch something. You're concerned that your water supply isn't up to EEC standards, and that the electricity pylons over your house might increase your risk of leukaemia, and you're worried about inconsistent labelling of GM food. You are certain that every dark skin blemish is a melanoma.

You present to the doctor with a mole/blemish, desperate for reassurance that it isn't cancer. Can the doctor be certain? How can they be certain? Can they put their hand on their heart and say that this isn't cancer? You then go through the various parts of your body that are worrying you and demand a total body scan to put your mind at rest. Try to really pin the doctor down on issues of certainty. Don't let them off the hook. How can they be sure? ('Could all this worrying I'm doing give me cancer?!')

You are not 'mad.' However, you have become unduly concerned about your health, which is becoming close to an obsession. You should come over as the 'informed worried (very worried) well' rather than as a crank. Having said that, some of your information is suspect and most of your conclusions are to some extent irrational.

*You will be given a Heath Education Authority booklet as a prop **on the day**. Point to the lists, etc. in it and ask awkward questions (e.g. 'It says here that diet may be a factor – which foods should I avoid?).*

If you have Internet access, please feel free to do a quick search and bring in any examples of information that might be useful in the consultation.

Comments

This scenario is of great value for two main reasons. First, the patient may appear a slightly bizarre individual and will consequently sometimes come close to reducing the student and the audience to giggles. This is, in one sense, the simplest way to help students to understand the need to take people seriously. When the role player judges this precisely and correctly, the way that her fear has closed in on her and deprived her of the opportunity to live well will shine through the superficial eccentricity of her compulsions, but it does not shine through with complete clarity.

Secondly, the role player has the perfect setting in which to press the doctor on the matter of risk, and in this sense the scenario raises the issue of how to discuss risk and certainty, as in fact many scenarios readily do. In this case, the patient is quite likely to say 'Do you know – yes, but do you really, really *know* – that I don't have cancer?' To which, of course, the utterly honest answer is 'No, I don't really, really know.' Or, even less helpfully, 'Well, it depends what you mean by "know" exactly.' However, although a full-on discussion of scientific epistemology is not exactly what is needed, epistemology is actually at the heart of the scenario, and a version of just these issues – what a doctor actually *means* by 'evidence' – needs to be presented.

The doctor will mean 'No, I don't have the clinical evidence – the evidence at least of negative findings – which would enable me to make this kind of absolute statement.' Beyond this, in fact, the doctor may feel 'No, I don't actually know. But come on, be reasonable about this.'

However, this is something that the patient cannot do, or cannot easily do.

Most participants are very good at taking patient-centredness seriously. They know it matters – indeed if they have a problem with it at all, it is often that they tend to take it for granted, and don't really question what it means. This scenario presents a challenge. What do we mean, in this case, by taking patient concerns seriously?

Well, at the most superficial level, it means not laughing at the patient. It also means understanding and empathising with her genuine anxiety. And it also means recognising that her family history of cancer is likely to be a major motivation for her behaviour, so that if we need to find something akin to a rationalisation of her attitude, there it is. However, this does not mean that we should value her opinion about risk as much as we value our own. Her beliefs are mistaken, and in that sense when she says 'I'm at terrible risk from cancer' she is exactly the same as the child who says in the student-centred classroom 'Berlin is the capital of Denmark.' Training encourages the teacher to take student views seriously, and the doctor to take patient views seriously. It talks much less about what to do when people are wrong.

No education can take place if the foundations are wrong. I can't learn successfully about the history of Berlin if I think it's in Denmark. No patient education can take place if the foundations are wrong. This is one of the most important and most basic of all communication messages. This patient can only be helped if her belief system is debunked. The trick is to do this with respect, and with an understanding that her anxiety is real, and that the self-imposed narrowness of the patient's life is a sad and unnecessary thing.

As always, the relationship needs to be placed on a sound therapeutic basis. That is, both parties have to work together to understand what the problem really is. True 'patient-centredness' in this context must spring in the first instance from a rejection of the patient's concerns.

Successful handling of the scenario implies successful questions. The student who merely sets out the *facts* about cancer ('The fact is that you're not at any real risk') has missed the Socratic point, and will be unheard, just as the student who says 'Don't be a bully' will be ignored. Elicitation is the likeliest route here – repeated, gentle and insistent – until the patient stops throwing up barricades, and begins to answer the questions.

So this aspect of the scenario is likely to begin something along the lines of 'May I say, I think, personally, that you worry too much. Do you think other people are as worried as you?'

To this and similar questions, the initial response is likely to be 'Oh, but they don't have the family problems I have . . .'

The trick of the scenario is to get the patient to the point of offering direct answers to direct questions – that is, to the point of playing the Socratic game: 'Do they worry as much as I do? No, they don't.'

Here is another individual who needs to be brought to the point of articulating unpleasant things about him- or herself.

Scenario for elicitation 2: What do you mean, I'm a bully?

Participant notes

You are an FY1 doctor (i.e. newly qualified) on your first rotation. You are enjoying the experience and engage well with your peers, who often come to you for professional but more often for personal advice.

Several members of your learning group have commented recently on the behaviour of Dr Joe/Josie Parks, another of the FY1 doctors, who they feel is becoming increasingly overbearing, often to the point of thoroughly intimidating the quieter members of the group.

You have all noticed how uncomfortable one particular FY1 doctor, Jack, has become. He is usually the butt of Joe/Josie Park's jokes, which are becoming increasingly unpleasant to be around. For example, Joe/Josie Parks has recently done the following in your presence:

- made regular jokes about Jack's tendency to blush (e.g. referring to him publicly as the 'Scarlet Pimpernel' or the 'Blushing Bride'). Some of these comments have been within earshot of consultants, patients and nursing staff – who have not, however, appeared surprised or attempted to take action
- undertaken an exaggerated impression that made you cringe, in which Jack's regional accent and home county were both belittled, leaving the group tongue-tied with embarrassment
- on one occasion mimed being drenched with water whenever Jack made a sudden movement (Jack sweats profusely when anxious, so you felt that this was particularly cruel)
- made exaggerated bored faces, rolled their eyes and yawned whenever Jack spoke, at a recent group case discussion exercise.

This constant barrage of insults is making Jack silent and even red-faced in front of the senior clinicians, and this is now clearly beginning to affect his assessments. Jack recently said to you that he was 'starting to dread each day' and had 'no idea' how to cope with Dr Parks.

You have been persuaded by several peers to try to intervene, by making Joe/Josie Parks aware of the effects of their behaviour, both on Jack and on the rest of the group. It has also crossed your mind that Joe/Josie could get into serious trouble if this matter comes to the attention of more diligent senior staff.

[Decide in advance with the facilitator whether you do or do not have permission to name individual peers when you give feedback.]

You approach Joe/Josie one morning, before the others arrive.

Role player's notes

You are Joe/Josie Parks, an FY1 doctor on your first rotation. You are confident, and a high achiever. You are enjoying professional life and relish the environment. Things have worked out well for you recently – at work you feel you have really 'caught the eye' of several senior figures. You regard yourself as popular with your peers. You enjoy your independence, but have no doubt that when the time is right you will have no problem settling down and having the perfect family.

In the mean time you see yourself as the life and soul of the party, and are very much at the hub of your team's social life. You suspect that events are often surreptitiously arranged around your availability, which supports your belief that people have a 'better time' when you are involved. You consider yourself to be an amusing person, and are always ready to crack a joke. This is often at the expense of others, but you've never regarded this as inappropriate – people can crack jokes at your expense if they like, obviously so long as they remember that you'll be dishing out some pretty sharp responses! Hey, everyone needs to laugh at themselves occasionally, and you are, after all, a very talented impersonator . . .

At the moment you find yourself regularly joking about Jack, a fellow FY1. His unfortunate mannerisms and personal habits make good material, and your witty impressions of him are, you believe, highly entertaining. Jack blushes a lot so jokes about his appearance come easily. He also has a habit of sweating profusely when anxious, which you have made fun of several times in a light-hearted sketch in which you mime being sprayed with water as he moves past you. He also has a marked regional accent which makes for good jokes about his home county. Your perception is that your peers find this as amusing as you do. The jokes described above typically happen on or just after ward rounds. You see this use of humour as therapeutic – for example, in helping the more uptight members of the group to relax in often pressured situations with demanding consultants and registrars.

You are not aware that your behaviour may be becoming offensive to either Jack or your other colleagues. In fact you even asked Jack if he was OK recently, after you had embarrassed him in a recent case discussion exercise by pulling bored faces. You didn't think he seemed too upset – he certainly didn't indicate to you in any way that the leg pulling was upsetting.

Your other thought is that 'having a bit of a laugh' might help to bring Jack out of his shell. Although you perceive him as bit of a wimp, you also think he could 'toughen up' with the right treatment. It has never crossed your mind that your 'treatment' might be doing more harm than good.

You will therefore be very surprised to hear that your peers are uncomfortable with your attitude and behaviour. Surely they're not serious? Why is everyone 'tip-toeing' around Jack? If he wants to be a doctor, surely he should stand on his own two feet and not need to have his hand held by others in the group?

If very well handled you might at least begin to make the link between this feedback and bullying. You might also share with a sensitive colleague the fact that you yourself were the butt of everyone's jokes at boarding school (which you hated), but that the experience 'gave you backbone' and 'made you the person you are today.' Actually it was humiliating in the extreme at times, so a very perceptive learner might be able to pick up on this and make links with the way Jack is feeling.

Comments

One of the more difficult aspects of writing role-play scenarios is that there is no prior reality to draw on. It's hard to begin a scenario with 'You have known your next patient for many years . . .' because that presupposes a relationship built up over those years, shared memories of previous interactions, and so on. It's simplest, but not always possible, to build the scenario so that this encounter, today, is the first meeting between the participants. Nothing relevant has happened previously, offstage.

However, if this is not possible, it makes sense to try to have the important previous events within the role player's control, rather than under the student's control. Here, clearly, a lot will rest on what was actually said, and what actually happened between the role player (as the bully) and Jack (the more diffident young doctor). It's important that Joe/Josie *is* to some extent a bully – that there is a case to answer – and therefore it's clearly important that the role player has thought this through in their own mind.

The learner's task here is to help Joe/Josie towards a moment of self-awareness. The techniques which are at stake are in essence those of the classroom, and appropriate in such circumstances as teaching, therefore – or role-play facilitation – and also in appraisals, and in any setting where giving negative feedback is likely to be an issue.

In essence this means the use of questions. In fact, if the role play is done badly, it will often mean that the participant has in effect harangued the role player: 'You mustn't make jokes at other people's expense . . .' If it is done well, the moment of insight – the apprehension that bullying has taken place – will come from the role player, not from the participant. The questioning will lead the role player ineluctably to what, as Socrates would say, they already know. The successful dialogue will take the following kind of shape:

- What actually happened?
- What was the response of those who overheard this incident/these incidents?
- Why do you think they found it funny? What evidence is there of this?
- What was Jack's response?
- Are you sure Jack found it funny? What evidence is there of this?
- If I told you people were concerned about your treatment of Jack, would you be surprised?
- Why do you think people are concerned?

The exact questions that are asked will depend on the level of insight that the role player offers. As we saw with Gerry Parker, because scenarios are not intended to be realistic, it is likely that the role player will bluster defensively for rather longer than might be typical, to give the learner practice in this type of language, and more exposure to the kind of defensive barriers that people throw up around themselves when they have been caught out.

Nevertheless, the fairly gentle and indirect questioning illustrated above is probably going to be enough for Jack to get the point. And accompanying this, there are elements of meta-discourse (that is, language which talks about the process of interaction) which can be used, and into which the insightful listener will buy. This includes:

1   ordinary signalling moves: 'I want to talk about a couple of things with you. First, . . . secondly . . .', 'Let's just explore that . . .'
2   comments on how things are going: 'Well, you've made that point quite forcefully already, perhaps . . .', 'Perhaps I didn't explain that too well . . . let me try again . . .'

This leaves us, as is so often the case, with the problem of the person who lacks insight. Here, we might want to say, the rule is that the less insight the person has, the more directness is necessary. And this, as you will probably have immediately observed, is a difficulty. If we are saying, as most people would want to say, that in general it's better for participants to work things through for themselves, and reach their own understanding (to internalise learning, in the fashionable term, in their own way), it's something of a problem to maintain also that sometimes we cannot afford this kind of indirectness. With weak participants above all, who most need help, surely we should strive to teach them in the manner in which we claim to believe. This, as Socrates might happily point out, is a contradiction revealed.

There are some possible answers, none of which are entirely satisfactory, and they can profitably be discussed in the context of this scenario.

1   The rule with any individual is to be as gentle as is compatible with Joe/Josie understanding the message. In other words, what is blunt to the individual with insight is gentle to the person without it, and will serve the same two functions of saving face and telling the truth.
2   Some people, in the end, can't be taught (or at any rate, can't be told about their problems). Their defensive barrier is too high – and therefore the psychological cost of facing the truth may be too great – for anyone to penetrate. Alternatively, they may appear to be very concrete thinkers, and seem unable to think at a reflective level. The issue with such people is not therefore to help them to gain insight, so that they can change their attitudes and their behaviour, but to manage the wider situation, and put them into a position where their problems cause minimum disruption for others.
3   If you have to give instructions, you should do so. What matters in the end is

that the individual's patterns of behaviour change, because this is how others are protected. If the individual has no clear understanding of why they are being asked to behave differently, this is of relatively little consequence.

The discussion of these issues raises profound questions, which may or (more likely, unless a lot of time is available) may not get discussed. For case 1 above, these concern the need for the good communicator in this quasi-teaching role to have insight him- or herself – an awareness of what the other person is picking up, and what they are not picking up. And, as a consequence, for the good teacher or communicator to have a range of styles at their disposal, which can be flexibly deployed as necessary. In case 2, what is it we mean by saying (or dismissing) some people as 'too concrete' in their thinking, or 'insufficiently intelligent', or just, broadly, 'lacking in insight'? And in case 3, there are issues of behaviour and attitude, or surface and depth (as these terms were used in *Language and Clinical Communication*).

Reference

1 Piaget J. Some aspects of operations. In: Piers MW, editor. *Play and Development: a symposium.* New York: Norton and Co.; 1972. p. 27.

CHAPTER 7

The basic scenario

John Skelton and Connie Wiskin

> Only through communication can human life hold meaning.
>
> (P Freire, *The Pedagogy of the Oppressed*[1])

Introduction

At this stage, let us look at a single, simple scenario for beginners. Year 1 students of a range of health professions can work with it, or with slight variations of it. It goes without saying that this scenario has the same potential for expansion as the scenarios mentioned earlier, but it was originally designed for the larger groups, and more tentative participants, discussed below.

Basic scenario: The bad back, the bad boss and the difficult in-law

Participant notes

You are a GP, and you are about to meet Robyn Taylor for the first time. Although she has been registered for many years, you observe that she has not attended for the last five years. There is no history of note.

Role player's notes

You are Robyn Taylor, a married librarian. You enjoy your work, and feel part of the team.

You have two worries.

First, you periodically experience back pain. There is no pattern, and you manage the pain by taking painkillers and relaxing at home for a week or two.

Your mother suffered similarly, and 'just got on with it', believing, like you, that doctor time is sacred. You have therefore never consulted a doctor about this problem. You are slightly in awe of health professionals. The pain is now severe.

Your former boss was sympathetic about illness absence, allowing you to 'make the time up' or turning a blind eye. However, he recently retired, and the new manager has made it clear that 'slacking' will not be tolerated. You are worried about his reaction. Worse still, you overhead him saying that previously he's had to manage malingerers who were always acting up 'back pain' and 'family troubles' to avoid hard work. A colleague has suggested that you should obtain a sick-note.

Secondly, your husband was born in Hong Kong, although he has lived in the UK for many years. An elderly relative of his has recently moved in, as her previous carer has taken a demanding job which involves a lot of travel. The relative has limited mobility, due to arthritis. You find that helping them in and out of chairs and bed is even tougher with the back pain. Your husband helps when he can during the day, but he works as a chef at a leading Chinese restaurant in the city centre, and is therefore away most evenings, leaving you alone as sole carer.

Backache aside, you worry how you will cope with this situation. There was uneasiness on both sides of the family about your marriage at first, and this has never completely disappeared (there was a dispute – one of many – about you retaining your maiden name of 'Taylor', rather than taking on your husband's name). You do your best to get on with your husband's relative, but she speaks little English and you speak less Cantonese, so it's difficult. And while she claims to want to move back because, as she says rather hurtfully, 'my daughters will look after me properly', you have seen little effort to facilitate this. You fear that the current 'temporary' arrangement could become permanent. The relatives in Hong Kong are stalling, and your husband (who is kind, passive, and preoccupied with the business, in which he has a financial stake) is reluctant to get involved in family politics. The relative has multiple health needs, but refuses to register with a local western doctor. She has told your husband that your doctors won't understand her as well as her previous doctor did (he was ethnic Chinese, in a western-style practice, but with an interest in Chinese medicine).

Communication is difficult, and without your husband to translate, you struggle at home. Can the doctor suggest a Cantonese-speaking doctor, at the very least?

Comments

The obvious reason why this scenario is appropriate for near beginners is the lack of clinical knowledge that is necessary in order to conduct it at some level of competence. Because there is little or no knowledge on which to base clinical advice (indeed, participants should be actively discouraged from guessing the correct advice), there is very little advice to be given, but this doesn't really matter. The aim of this scenario is to find out why the patient has come to the doctor today – a phrase which can itself, of course, be played with various emphases – as a general enquiry, or with the stress on 'why today?'

There are a number of possible successful methodologies, and the reader may well be able to think of others in addition to those listed below. Here is a suggested lesson plan, assuming a group of 15–20 students (larger than the ideal, which is probably more like 4–6, but curriculum pressure often demands larger groups). This approach relies on the role player being able to present two different versions of the scenario – one in which the patient's main worry is the stigma of claiming to have a problem which is associated with malingerers, and which may have implications for their present problem, and the other in which the patient is more concerned with the family repercussions.

Lesson plan

Aim of lesson:
1. To familiarise students with the concept of role play
2. To raise student awareness of 'communication' as a necessary area of expertise
3. To introduce basic skills such as open/closed questions, expressions of empathy, and checking skills
4. To allow students to work in a setting which exemplifies stigma and cross-cultural issues

Stage 1: Introduction

Welcome	2 minutes
Explanation of lesson aims	3 minutes
Explanation of procedures/setting class rules	5 minutes

Stage 2: Introduction of scenario

Read scenario   2 minutes

Questions: 'Why do people go to the doctor?' (lay referral, etc.), 'What common first presentations are there?' (headaches, flu, etc.), 'This patient suffers from backache – what does that mean?', 'Is backache common?', 'Is backache a medical problem?', etc.

8 minutes

Stage 3: Round-robin questions

> Throughout, students play the part of medical students (i.e. they don't aim to imitate doctors).
>
> Students remain seated as they are, in a horseshoe-shaped arrangement. The role player faces them. Students ask questions round the class. The role player responds in line with Version 1 of the scenario, concentrating on the issue of stigma and fear of unemployment ('Oh, the family's a nuisance, but that's not the main thing . . .')
>
> 10 minutes

Stage 4: Feedback

> What kind of questions seemed to work? What conclusions did you reach about the patient? What advice would you give the patient?
>
> 10 minutes

Stage 5: Group work

> Students are divided into two groups, A and B.
>
> 'Next, we'll see the same scenario, but with the role player more concerned about family issues. In your groups, suggest questions to ask.'
>
> 10 minutes

Stage 6: One-to-one role play, with Group A

> 'Three of you will talk to the patient, one after the other, with the second student picking up the conversation where the first has left off, and so on. The other three will make notes to provide feedback later.'
>
> Students may ask for a 'Time out' within the group, to seek help. The teacher reserves the right to call for time out, to draw attention to specific issues, and to give direct feedback to students.
>
> 15 minutes

Stage 7: Repeat for Group B

> 15 minutes

Stage 8: Feedback within groups (5 minutes for each group)

> 10 minutes

This gives a session of 90 minutes (exactly the same lesson could easily be expanded) working with two versions of a single role play, and a single role player. If well handled, and with an enthusiastic group of participants – which is a reasonable assumption – this will seem challenging and interesting. Altering a scenario of this kind more substantially (for example, by giving the patient two different jobs for the two different versions, and therefore probably altering such things as the husband's job, and the educational background of both parties, etc.) will offer more variation in the lesson, which may well be an advantage, but will rely on the role player being able to change fairly quickly from one person to the other.

Preparation and follow-up lessons are probably more difficult in the health professions than they are elsewhere, given the normally very heavy timetable demands on students. With regard to the circumstances for which we wrote this scenario, it is designed to support the strand known as 'Medicine in Society', and also to complement the community-based attachment that students have in a primary care setting at the same time.

I have presented a 90-minute version of the scenario here in order to illustrate a range of possible approaches. The scenario will obviously work using a smaller number of approaches, and would take a shorter time as a result.

There are a number of fairly routine general points to make about this approach to the teaching of communication.

First, this scenario illustrates the general point discussed earlier, that there is a difference between what is *taught*, what is *learned* and what is *acquired*. This three-way distinction is built into the fabric of communication skills teaching. There will be some overt teaching points which the teacher wants to get across – these are some of the things which appear above as lesson aims. However, what the teacher aspires to deliver is not what the learner necessarily concentrates on, and in any case because of the different experiences that are brought to bear on the situation being explored, what is observed will be interpreted differently (perhaps in trivial ways, occasionally not) from person to person. And, beyond that, a great deal will be unconsciously acquired, through observation of all parties involved. This is also the nature of PBL, namely that control over the learner's learning is much less than in other types of curriculum – a fact which makes it more difficult, among other things, to be too specific about lesson aims.

Secondly, there is a very straightforward question to be answered. Given that these students are already meeting and talking to patients as part of their community-based attachment (and given the fact that communication skills courses usually run alongside the opportunity to meet 'real patients'), why bother with the administratively difficult and fairly expensive type of intervention that role play represents?

The usual answer to this question – and of course this is perfectly correct – is that role play offers the opportunity for honest and articulate feedback which patients do not offer, and that both the role play and the feedback take place in a safe environment. This remains the major justification for many people, but there are other reasons. One is that, by using role play, one can select what the student is exposed to, both in terms (obviously enough) of clinical content, and also in terms of overall difficulty. In this respect, any reasonably trained role player can make the same scenario more or less difficult as required. Another reason, a point made in an earlier chapter but not usually mentioned, is that role play is not designed to mirror reality.

The inauthentic parts of a play in the theatre include both the manipulation of events for aesthetic and dramatic effect, and the fact that everyone speaks without hesitating, mumbling, repeating themselves, and so on. As it happens, the hesitations and false starts of authentic speech are well captured in a role play, because it isn't scripted – but role plays, in the hands of a skilled role player, are full of the manipulations of an educator. It is the role player's task to bring the conversation to a series of cruxes, to offer the student the opportunity to practise in certain areas.

The most obvious cruxes we have seen to date are (with Mr Stafford, from the first of the rich context scenarios) how to express regret against the background of a complaint (and an understanding of the issues which surround this), and (with Gerry Parker) how to insist on the professional nature of the interaction (and a similar understanding of the issues here). It follows therefore that each scenario, over time, develops its own particular shape, or more precisely a number of shapes, depending on how the student handles it. And it follows from this that the feedback on offer will also develop a range of patterns.

Thirdly, all scenarios ultimately deal with the question 'What is it to be a doctor (or nurse, or whatever is relevant)?' That is, the most fundamental mechanics of the situation, in which the facilitator and audience are watching the role player and student, and in which the role player is both within and beyond the dialogue, participating and watching at the same time, and in which the participants are invited to reflect (to watch themselves retrospectively), all invite an exceptionally high degree of awareness of the process. In the case of the participant who is engaged in the role play, this means self-awareness. The creation and representation of the professional self are what is ultimately at stake.

Fourthly, giving students and others permission to stop and start the role play by calling for a time-out has one major disadvantage. A conversation, any conversation, is constructed between the participants. To halt and restart it artificially undermines the reality of the construct, perhaps in terms of believability (although as Dr Johnson once remarked scathingly, no one who is watching a play actually believes that what they see is 'real'), but more probably in terms of the language used to conduct the subsequent interaction. On the other hand, it has the obvious virtue with beginner students of giving them a resource if they get stuck, and also of involving spectators, who may feel more engaged because they have the opportunity to make a contribution. It has the further virtue of allowing the facilitator to invite speculation, with questions like 'OK, you've seen the patient, and she's begun to talk about her back pain – what words would you use to describe her?'

To which the answers might be clinical, or might pick up on the anxiety which is probably already on display, or might reflect on the patient's general presentation (for example, 'she seems a shy sort of person'). This in turn allows for a range of questions to do with evidence ('What did she do, exactly, that makes you think she's shy/anxious . . .?'), and also provides the opportunity to explore the extent to which participants are making, or jumping to, conclusions. For example, 'What kind of job do you think she might have?' is likely to elicit a range of responses ranging from 'We don't know yet, it could be anything' to the correct guess. To which perhaps the facilitator might respond 'Do you mean that shy people end up becoming librarians?'

This innocent sort of challenge opens up to students the relationship we have already looked at, between on the one hand the pattern making we must indulge in if we are not to try to reinterpret the world on a moment-by-moment basis, and on the other hand the kind of crass stereotype (librarians are shy) which is at the root of prejudice.

Fifthly, with students at the start of their professional career, there is a need to offer them a basic vocabulary if they are to reflect on communication. At first, this can be the vocabulary of the skills syllabus, and the distinction between open and closed questions is a likely starting point – except, alas, that it is a pretty shaky distinction.

There is a linguistic distinction between question types which offers an approximate parallel. This distinction is best known in its language teachers' guise, as a distinction between 'wh- questions' and 'yes/no questions.' The former are questions which start with a 'wh- word' such as *what, when, why, where,* or – annoyingly – *how.* The latter are questions which can be given a single-word response, *yes* or *no.* These questions start with the word *do, does, did, have, has, had,* etc. It's a standard teacher's trick to use a 'wh- question' to elicit longer answers from students, and it has its parallel in contemporary sports interviewing in the UK, when sports stars, not a famously articulate bunch of people on the whole, are not asked 'Are you pleased you won?', but rather 'How pleased are you that you've won?'

In clinical communication, however, 'wh- questions' tend to be regarded as closed, because they tend, it is said, to elicit short answers. Certainly they can be used for this purpose, in questions like 'When did you first notice the pain?' ('Last Tuesday, doctor'). However, this is by no means an invariable rule, and perhaps the shortness of the response is to do with factors like the doctor's approach – they ask a series of 'wh- questions' fairly quickly, for purely clinical reasons, to rule out some diagnoses and rule in others, for example. And in fact there is no formal description of a 'closed question.' The concept seems only to mean 'a question which elicits a short answer', and the definition is therefore narrowly circular. Still, the distinction itself – between short and long responses – is useful.

There is one other point to make about this particular scenario, and indeed any scenario in which there is an activity such as asking questions round the room. What is lost under these circumstances is the distinction, normal in real interaction, between certain aspects of what is best known as 'main' and 'subsidiary' discourse.[2] 'Main' discourse is, roughly, the main thrust of the argument – questions such as 'How long have you had the pain?', 'Do you associate it with any type of activity?', 'Is it there all the time, or is it more noticeable on certain occasions?' and the associated answers. Subsidiary discourse is, among other things, the language of support, empathy and the like which surrounds this – for example, 'It's there all the time? – Oh dear, that must be a nuisance for you', and so on. This kind of language doesn't survive the format. Students tend to go from one content question (one piece of main discourse) to the next.

The above lesson plan is for a group of 15 or so participants (and assumes two available teaching spaces, of course, for the group work). Often, however, people are working in even more straitened circumstances. Here is an example of the same scenario in different circumstances, which cost the host institution less.

Forum theatre

This is designed for groups of 60–100 participants.

For this exercise, you need a couple of role players who are able to do role play onstage – which clearly indicates that professional (or at any rate experienced amateur) actors are best, although experienced lecturers also tend to be capable of projecting basic scenarios well. One of these will take the patient's part, and the other will take the health professional's part. You also need a facilitator who is able to lead discussion with a large group – and, possibly, someone with a roving microphone to move among the audience.

Stage 1:   (led by facilitator)

'Here are some questions to consider. First, why do people go to the doctor? Second, what do you know about stigma? Third, what is a 'holistic' consultation? Think about these questions for a minute or two . . .'

'. . . OK? Right, any ideas?'

Ideas elicited from audience

5–10 minutes

Stage 2:   (led by facilitator)

'Now you're going to meet a patient and a health professional. Here is the patient . . . here is the doctor . . . (indicating role players).'

'Let me read you the scenario . . .' (facilitator reads scenario)

'OK?'

'Right – they're going to do the role play.'

'The health professional isn't necessarily on their best behaviour. As you watch, think about what they do well, and what they do badly.'

2–4 minutes

Stage 3:   Role play 1

The health professional undertakes the role play, but does it badly. If this is over the top, it ends up being funny, and is a good sensitisation exercise for complete beginners. For a group who are not complete beginners, hamming it up is a waste of time. The poor quality needs to be sufficiently subtle for the audience to think as they watch.

5–8 minutes

Stage 4:   Giving advice (led by facilitator)

'Any advice for our health professional? What was done well? What was done badly?'

Responses are elicited from the audience. The role player, in role, fields these comments: 'You mean I shouldn't have said . . .?' 'So you think it would be better if I . . .?'

7–15 minutes

Stage 5: Role play 2

The scenario is repeated. This can be done either simply from beginning to end, or with the role player stopping at various points to ask 'Was that better?'

7–15 minutes

Stage 6: Round-up (led by facilitator)

'So we've seen that the central issues in this scenario are . . .'

5–8 minutes

This gives a session of 30–60 minutes.

References

1 Freire P. *The Pedagogy of the Oppressed.* New York: Continuum; 1970.
2 Coulthard M, Montgomery M, editors. *Studies in Discourse Analysis.* London: Longman; 1981.

CHAPTER 8

Strange shadows

John Skelton and Connie Wiskin

What is your substance, whereof are you made,
That millions of strange shadows on you tend?
Since every one hath, every one, one shade,
And you, but one, can every shadow lend.

(William Shakespeare, Sonnet 53[1])

Introduction

The aim of this chapter is simply to offer the reader a range of scenarios, with minimal commentary, in the hope that he or she will follow through some of the thoughts and suggestions in previous chapters, and consider whether they might apply here as well.

Shakespeare's Sonnet 53 is in fact generally regarded as a piece of Neoplatonism – the idea is that, just as the Godhead infuses all of creation, so the lover sees the world infused with the presence of the beloved. However, it is also therefore a contemplation on the nature of human identity, and of how one perceives it. There are obvious risks of bathos in talking about Shakespeare and clinical communication in the same breath, but the question of who the patient actually is should always be present, even if it is merely an insistent whisper in the health professional's ear.

Scenario 1: After the revelation

Participant notes

You are a GP, and you are about to see Luke/Lucy Kirby. You haven't seen them before, but they are known to have mild cerebral palsy and come for regular check-ups and repeat prescriptions. They were prescribed baclofen 5 mg TDS as a muscle relaxant 6 months ago. They are not due for a review.

- Medical history: Wore a special shoe and a calliper as a child, and had childhood operations to stretch the Achilles tendon to correct gait.
- Physiotherapy and hydrotherapy from the ages of 4–16 years to strengthen muscles.
- Allergic to fur. Takes an over-the-counter antihistamine occasionally when exposed to the allergen.
- Drug history: Prescribed both oral and topical anti-spasmodics (muscle relaxants/anti-spasm medication).

Role player's notes

You are Luke/Lucy Kirby. You are single, though you have recently begun a relationship with a girlfriend/boyfriend, and you work in a call centre (as a travel adviser).

You have a mild form of cerebral palsy (CP) which has caused muscle weakness on the right side of your body. You walk with a slight limp and your right hand 'isn't much use.' This has not been a problem at work, as the phones have headsets and you type well with your left hand.

The type of CP that you have is spastic hemiplegia. Your brain was probably damaged by lack of oxygen at birth, which means that the signals your brain gives to the right side of your body aren't as effective as the ones that it gives to the left side. The right-side muscles are tight and stiff, weaker than those on the left side, and prone to spasm.

These spasms/cramps can be frequent and painful. Six months ago you were prescribed baclofen 5 mg TDS as a muscle relaxant, which had positive effects, leaving you spasm free. This was a major relief, enabling you to thrive professionally and gain confidence socially.

Three weeks ago you stopped your medication, after what you can only describe as 'a religious experience.'

You have always been a 'spiritual' person but have never followed a formal religion. Your parents believed in God but were not churchgoers. Your father died in an accident when you were a child, and you and your mother remain close.

A few months ago your mother confided that she had had a 'vision' in a compelling dream that inspired her to stop taking her arthritis medication. She reported that in the vision she was told to 'believe in prayer, and trust what nature has provided.' You were sceptical at first, but the difference has been remarkable. Astonishingly, she is pain-free and seems to have better use of her joints than she has had for years.

Three weeks ago you had the same dream, several times. You are certain that the message was to turn to prayer, to nature and away from chemicals. You know how this might sound, and you acknowledge that a few weeks ago you would have struggled to believe it.

However, you have not experienced dramatic improvements, and discomfort from the CP is returning. You have noticed that some things have eased without drugs (a headache vanished within minutes of prayer, and sneezing when exposed to animals stopped when you used the same method), but you have not been so lucky with the CP. You interpret this as being 'tested.'

The cramps are creeping back, but you feel that it would be *deeply wrong* to restart the tablets, given the privilege of the vision. You find working uncomfortable, and your girlfriend/boyfriend is worried. They have been supportive of your beliefs, but have suggested that you ask a doctor about alternatives (e.g. a faith healer).

Today you hope to (a) state for your patient notes that you no longer accept 'man-made' medicines, and (b) ask for a 'natural' alternative to tide you over until the effects of prayer kick in. You pride yourself on not letting illness affect your life. Your parents wanted you to be 'normal', and you are keen not to be regarded as disabled.

You are composed and intelligent and do not hold any outrageous views. The revelation has simply prompted a change in health beliefs. You expect to be taken seriously.

Comments

Different people believe different things. What matters here is the extent to which the patient is taken seriously (see earlier scenarios), and the way in which the patient's health beliefs are taken up – if they are (and if they aren't, why not) – and used when negotiating a management plan.

It was suggested in *Language and Clinical Communication* (and earlier, p. 52) that in addition to what we may these days describe as the traditional 'triaxial' view of the consultation (i.e. that it consists of biological, social and psychological axes), we might add an ethical and interpersonal axis – together perhaps with others, such as the spiritual axis which is clearly relevant here.

This is also evidently a scenario where the ethical axis is of considerable importance and, with regard to the interpersonal issues, there is scope for the participant perhaps to say 'I know nothing about faith healers', and also perhaps to say 'I think they're ineffectual' without losing the patient's trust, and without damaging the doctor–patient relationship.

This scenario, in the end, balances uneasily between the view (one might say – rather unfairly – the quasi-constructionist view) that everyone makes their own reality and that no one's reality is 'truer' than anyone else's, and on the other hand the view that there are true things and untrue things. And that, when it comes to medicine, the doctor is more likely to know the true things than the patient.

Scenario 2: Admission demand

Participant notes

Note: If you are bi- or multilingual please inform the facilitator before undertaking the scenario, as it is designed to offer the challenge of not having a language in common with your patient.

You are a doctor working in Accident and Emergency at a busy city hospital (grade as appropriate). It is Saturday evening.

Your patient, Mrs Seeta Malik, has attended because her son Asad (aged 18 months) has developed a rash on his arm. Mrs Malik initially arrived with two female relatives, and another female child aged about 8 years. You established that in the absence of her husband, who is at work, these relatives (her husband's sisters) have come to offer transport and moral support. It seems also that Asad was seen first by a nurse, for triaging purposes, but the nurse, flustered by a relative whom she found demanding, has sent Asad on to you, to be on the safe side.

Mrs Malik's English is limited, so one of the relatives acted as a lay interpreter while you took a history and performed a thorough examination of the child. The boy had no additional symptoms, and the rash appeared to be a mild allergic reaction. There were no sinister or worrying findings. You reassured the relatives that it was fortunately unlikely to be anything serious, you prescribed a topical cream to alleviate the itching, and you recommended that the rash should be monitored, with a trip to the GP advisable on Monday if it was still present. *Discuss with the group any other advice you might have given before commencing the role play.*

At this point Asad began to cry, and after an 'agitated-sounding' conversation between the women present (in which you were not included) one of the female relatives left with Asad and the other child, leaving Mrs Malik and her 'interpreter' in the cubicle. The interpreter says 'We will not go.'

The scenario starts at this point. The role player will lead in.

Note: This scenario can be modified to suit any nationality of patient, and can also be undertaken as managing a patient who has some English and does not have a lay interpreter present, or who is using a professional medical interpreter.

Role players' notes

You are Mrs Seeta Malik and her sister-in-law Nasrin. You have come to Accident and Emergency on Saturday evening worried about a rash which has appeared on the arm of Seeta's son Asad.

In addition to Nasrin, who is here to translate, another sister-in-law and her 8-year-old daughter also came to Accident and Emergency. The additional relative gave them a lift in her car, bringing her daughter along as well to avoid having to arrange childcare.

Seeta

You are married to a British citizen and you arrived in the UK two years ago, already pregnant with Asad. You worked in a jewellery store in India before your marriage, but a combination of being a mother and having limited English language skills has so far deterred you from thinking about employment in the UK. Your husband is a train driver so, as is the case tonight, he is sometimes away in the evenings. You are very close to him, and you wish that he was here tonight to share the experience. He is proving an excellent father, and tonight you are determined to protect your son's interests on behalf of both of you.

You are very worried, and you are not convinced by the doctor's explanation. Nasrin translated a lot of questions about Asad's health, and you responded truthfully that he had no other symptoms. However, surely the very visible rash is enough to warrant concern? Nasrin said the doctor had said that 'It was not serious, use cream and phone the GP later.' Your interpretation of this is that the doctor has trivialised your worries. How can any alien marks on a baby be 'not serious'?

To confound matters you remember that in India once a cousin's baby was dismissed by a hospital and died a few days later. You were young when this happened and you don't recall the medical details, but you do remember that the child was 'red.'

You want an admission and overnight monitoring, ideally from a 'special baby doctor.' During an emotive discussion with your two sisters-in-law you decide between you not to be 'fobbed off.' Nasrin stays with you for the sit-in, while your other relative takes a bawling Asad for a walk and removes her own little girl from earshot. You don't know the NHS rules, but you know your rights as a mother. You decide to stay for as long as it takes.

Nasrin

You are close to your family, and keen to help. You have lived in the UK for 10 years longer than Seeta, and have more developed language skills. Unlike Seeta you work – at a nursery at your community centre. You do not have children yet (although you plan to), but still consider yourself something of an 'expert' because of your job. Although you are 'good with children', the reality is that you have no specialist experience, but this doesn't prevent you from having opinions. You are fond of saying things like 'In my experience you can't be too careful with children' and 'In my job we have to take our responsibility seriously', and will probably challenge the doctor with this.

Your translation is reasonable. You don't deliberately set out to mislead, but you do have a habit of over-summarising. You are unlikely to challenge Seeta's desire to stay put in the hospital. Although you have more understanding of the NHS than her, you certainly don't want to be blamed if you have any identifiable part in her 'going home too early and things going wrong.'

You may show your support by saying to the doctor things like 'She knows her human rights', 'She's a good mother' and 'You and me, doctor, we can work together to protect Asad.' Start the scenario with 'Doctor, we will not go.'

In short, both of you are determined to stay at least the night for safety's sake. You want a cot to be brought to Accident and Emergency to keep the baby comfortable while his ward place is arranged. You have packed bags with belongings for all three of you ready in the car in anticipation of an admission.

Reassurance and risk explanation are required. The reaction probably stems from a first-time mother's fear and desire to protect her child. Asad was playing at a friend's home earlier, he crawled in the garden and played with their pets, so exposure to an allergic reaction was not impossible. However, neither of you are likely to make this connection unsupported.

Comments

This has the potential to be either a difficult scenario or a relatively easy one, depending on how determined Seeta is, how good the language skills of both parties are, and how good Nasrin's translation skills are. Any interaction where there is more than one lay participant is potentially a problem, and the issues are greatly complicated by the question of translation.

The main themes are therefore going to cluster round:

■ developing skills in briefing and communicating with a lay (or professional) interpreter, including understanding the implications of this three-way dialogue

■ explaining and contextualising clinical risk – here, for example, meningitis and allergic symptoms

■ communicating effectively with patients who appear to challenge the doctor's diagnosis and, by implication, his or her expertise. This includes recognising (and acknowledging) fear

- maintaining confidentiality in scenarios where immediate and extended family members may be present
- appropriately managing NHS resources – what the NHS can and cannot do, and what it is reasonable and unreasonable to expect. Here, if poorly handled, the family might try to gain admission to, for example, unauthorised areas.

Scenario 3: Talking about death and dying

Participant notes

Patrick/Patricia Coles was diagnosed with skin cancer three years ago. An operation appeared to be successful in the short term, but a month ago the cancer returned (it had spread to the liver). A consultant's report confirmed that the cancer was inoperable. The patient has been referred to a hospice doctor. You have not met Patrick/Patricia before.

Agree the setting in advance. The healthcare professional role can be any relevant member of the primary or secondary care team. The scenario can be set at home (e.g. during a specialist nurse home visit).

Role player's notes

You are Patrick/Patricia Coles. A month ago you developed stomach pain. It has since been discovered that your skin cancer (which was operated on successfully three years ago) has returned and spread to your liver. The consultant has explained that there is no intervention for this, and that you will soon see a hospice doctor who will 'keep you comfortable.' You have made the most of the last three years, and are reconciled to the outcome.

However, you would like to know what dying from cancer is likely to be like.

You also know very little about your pending hospice care. In your limited experience, a hospice equates with 'the end.'

Your brother and sister do not yet know that the cancer has returned, and that it is incurable. How much should you tell them? Should you hide the truth to protect them from distress? Your partner has been informed, and has been wonderful. Both of your parents died in old age.

You suspect that you contracted cancer from sunbed overuse, and you feel 'a bit damn stupid' now. You wonder if the healthcare professional thinks the same thing, and how other healthcare professionals might react to 'self-inflicted' cancer.

Comments

The main themes that are likely to arise are listed below, although they will vary in individual significance from one participant to another, and from less experienced to more experienced participants. This scenario can be used for basic communication skills training. It raises the topic of death, obviously enough, without being a traditional 'breaking bad news' scenario, and in that sense is useful for helping less experienced students or healthcare professionals to find the courage and the language to relax and seek to be of genuine assistance.

Some of the main themes include:

- conversing sensitively, but honestly, when hope is gone. Making judicious language choices when talking about death (how, when, why . . .?)
- managing different patients' reactions to unwelcome news
- recognising and normalising guilt reactions and public/professional attitudes towards 'self-inflicted' illness
- facilitating dialogue using communication and counselling skills
- involving colleagues – teamwork (including support) and service provision during the end-of-life journey for the patient, carer and healthcare professional.

Scenario 4: My grandson's secret

Participant notes

You are a GP or practice nurse. You are about to meet Mr Alec/Mrs Alice Styles. Mr/Mrs Styles is a long-term widower/widow who has partial responsibility for the care of their teenage grandson Jason Styles, aged 14. You last saw Mr/Mrs Styles six months ago when Jason had a heat rash.

Role player's notes

You are Mrs Alice/Mr Alec Styles, a widow/widower with a teenage grandson, Jason, aged 14. Your daughter (a factory worker) lives nearby. She is a single mother, and you have always shared the childcare, taking early retirement from your cleaning job to help her when she gave birth at the age of 15.

Recently, while tidying Jason's room at your house, you were horrified to discover a box containing condoms and what looked like 'rolled up' cigarettes.

You have lost sleep over this, but have no idea what to do. You have not discussed the matter with your daughter. You love her, but acknowledge that she can be 'a bit unstable.' She suffers from mood swings and is prone to what you think of as 'irrational' tempers, which confuse Jason.

You did not discuss sex openly during your own marriage, nor did you discuss it with your daughter. You wonder if this is why she ended up in such a mess, and you would be devastated if Jason's life was similarly ruined. This time you want to get it right.

Jason's father (long gone) was a 'rough sort.' Jason has recently mentioned the possibility of trying to find him – something that you've actively discouraged. In general, Jason is a decent kid. Recently, though, he has become 'moodier' and more withdrawn, and you're unsure of the suitability of his 'crowd.'

You've seen horror stories in the media about the terrible fates that befall teenagers these days. What if Jason gets a disease like AIDS, or ends up being a father now? What if he is already addicted to cigarettes . . . or worse. You've heard that drugs 'kill' brain cells. Your mind is in overdrive.

You know that it is your duty to tackle all of this, but you want 'proper information' and advice on how to do it. Better still, you would like the healthcare professional to offer to speak to Jason. You feel awkward about discussing sensitive subjects, and will need help getting started.

Comments

The focus of this scenario is likely to be helping Mr/Mrs Styles to be articulate, by doing many or most of the following things:

- acknowledging and managing patient anxiety by listening, prompting and effective listening
- talking confidently, comfortably, without prejudice and clearly about potentially sensitive subjects such as addiction, sex and sexuality
- exploring and explaining adolescent behaviour – helping the patient to understand what is typical and what may not be
- managing resources – considering what aspects of this family's past and current history might be legitimised as 'medical' problems; thinking about whether aspects outside these boundaries remain within the doctor's remit
- working with age diversity (e.g. what modifications might the healthcare professional make – or not make – if talking to a teenager as opposed to a grandparent?); emphasising the need for flexibility.

Scenario 5: Working with Terry

Participant notes

You are a general dental practitioner. Alex Davies is the parent/carer of Terry, a patient in their early twenties with a learning disability. You have just examined Terry for the first time.

Clinical examination findings: Extensive caries in the four first permanent molars. Two teeth can be saved and filled, but the other two require extraction. The treatment requires three visits, one each for the extractions and a further one for the fillings. Because of complications relating to heart problems, and following the current trend towards the use of local anaesthetic, you are not prepared to use general anaesthetic for this procedure. *(Note: more experienced clinicians may wish to negotiate their own treatment plan.)*

Alex has dominated throughout the clinical examination, so you are unsure how articulate Terry is.

The role play begins after the examination. Explain the treatment plan to Alex and Terry, and obtain appropriate consent. You also need to tackle the issue of oral care. There is considerable evidence of neglect.

Role players' notes

You are Alex Davies and Terry. Alex is Terry's parent/carer. Terry is an adult with a learning disability. The dentist will explain the findings of an examination that has just taken place.

Alex will be unhappy about the treatment prescribed by the dentist. He/she is very protective and wants Terry to be given a general anaesthetic. He/she also believes that it will be less stressful for Terry to have all the work done 'in one go' while unconscious, instead of submitting to several visit for different things to be done with local anaesthetics.

In addition, Alex is (mistakenly) convinced that Terry is frightened of needles. Alex thinks that, with little experience of dentists, Terry will not cope with the recommended treatment plan.

Alex may be defensive because he/she doesn't resist Terry's predilection for sweets. Alex's level of knowledge about oral hygiene is not high – he/she may be suspicious that the dentist is trying to prolong the procedure for financial gain. Alex is over-protective and overbearing if not checked. If Terry is given an opportunity to contribute, it will be revealed that he/she *is* capable of some communication and judgement (the level of which is to be agreed with the facilitators).

Comments

Acknowledging Terry's right to be treated normally is not usually a problem in the abstract. The difficulty lies in finding ways to actually successfully relate to him, as one might expect. There is also the point, incidentally, that participants and observers often bend over backwards to indicate their lack of prejudice, and their deep appreciation of Terry as a person – in a way which can often sound anxiously patronising. The matter-of-fact tone which is so typical of the good practitioner in difficult circumstances is often harder to find than participants expect.

Typical main themes might be as follows, again with different emphases at different levels of experience:

■ including everyone – in this case the extent to which the learner managed to involve Terry in the conversation, and the impact of this on the three-way dynamic

- obtaining (informed) consent. This is a difficult area, and it largely relies on the judgement of the dentist in assessing competence. The capacity to make an assessment in this case will depend on the extent to which Terry was involved
- strategies for communicating with patients with learning difficulties
- understanding and explaining the concept of best interest. Reassuring all parties that the recommended course of action was in the best interests of the patient
- giving potentially awkward feedback on personal hygiene. How successfully did the learner deal with the issue of neglected oral care?

Scenario 6: Fear of theatre

Participant notes

You are a hospital doctor (grade as appropriate).

Liam/Leanne Wheeler is in for a scheduled operation for repair of an inguinal hernia later this afternoon. On admission earlier today Liam/Leanne was chatting to their partner and appeared relaxed. When you return to the ward the partner has left. Liam/Leanne asks for a 'quick private word' in a side room.

Role player's notes

You are Liam/Leanne Wheeler. You are in hospital for a hernia repair later today (there is a swelling in the groin, not life-threatening, but uncomfortable and needing repair).

You have been admitted to a surgical ward. Your partner has gone home, and since then you have become increasingly agitated about what lies ahead.

You have approached the operation bravely, both as a coping strategy for yourself, and to minimise worry for your partner. You don't like to 'make a fuss.'

In fact, you are very anxious. This is not so much about the necessity for the procedure as about the prospect of being in theatre. The idea of 'going under' is one you are finding particularly difficult to cope with.

You met the anaesthetist earlier on the ward, and he asked questions about your general health. Although he was personable, he was quite difficult to understand (his first language was not English). He asked you whether you had any questions, and while several came to mind, you couldn't quite bring yourself to admit to your anxieties. After all, the other patients appeared unconcerned.

You now regret not speaking up. You have just noticed a doctor who smiled at you earlier, so you decide to take the plunge and ask for a chat.

The following things are on your mind:

- You read a horrific article in a newspaper about a person who had an operation and felt every cut, but couldn't cry out.
- You wonder what training anaesthetists have. Is it safe to put your life in their hands?
- You have no idea what happens in theatre. For example, how many people will be watching? Will students be practising things on you?
- The thought of being 'displayed' naked is mortifying.
- Are you 'normal' or over-reacting?

Once you are in full flow you are known to go on a bit . . .

Comments

This scenario is essentially about how fear surfaces, and how healthcare professionals should seek to understand it and alleviate it.

Typical main themes might include the following:

- explaining knowledge (or not) of theatre procedures, and normalising the patient's reaction to the prospect of going there
- recognising strong emotions and showing empathy
- effectively managing time during the interview, taking control where necessary with a very talkative patient, and considering priorities
- educating the patient about a colleague's competence and qualifications (in this case explaining what an anaesthetist is, but leading on to a wider discussion of patient perceptions of staff on different teams in the hospital hierarchy)
- responding to a media story – managing the relationship between media representations of medics and the medical world, and patient expectations of the health services.

Reference

1 Shakespeare W. Sonnet 53. In: Jowett J, Montgomery W, Taylor G, Wells S, editors. *The Oxford Shakespeare: the complete works.* 2nd ed. Oxford: Oxford University Press; 2005. p. 785.

CHAPTER 9

Notes on the game of writing scientific text

. . . my present work shall be but to divert and recreate, as well as excite you by the delivery of matters of fact, such as you may for the most part try with much *ease*, and possibly not without some *delight*: And lest you should expect any thing of Elaborate or Methodical in what you will meet with here, I must confess to you before-hand, that the seasons I was wont to chuse to devise and try Experiments about Colours, were those daies, wherein having taken Physick, and finding my self as unfit to speculate, as unwilling to be altogether idle, I chose this diversion, as a kind of Mean betwixt the one and the other . . .

. . . Yea, that you may not think mee too reserv'd, or look upon an Enquiry made up of meer Narratives, as somewhat jejune, [I] am content to *premise* a few considerations, that now offer themselves to my thoughts, which relate in a more general way, either to the Nature of Colours, or to the study of it . . . And if I can invite Ingenious men to undertake such Tasks, I doubt not but the Curious will quickly obtain a better Account of Colours, than as yet we have, since in our Method the Theorical part of the Enquiry being attended, and as it were interwoven with the Historical, whatever becomes of the disputable Conjectures, the Philosophy of Colours will be promoted by the indisputable Experiments.

(Robert Boyle, *Experiments and considerations touching colours*[1])

Introduction

The last of the language games I want to discuss is the game of academic writing, particularly writing for publication. I wish to do so partly because I believe it's a helpful way to assist people over the initial barriers which rise forbiddingly between them and an understanding of the clinical literature. People – their teachers, their colleagues, their bosses – expect them to read so that they can keep up professionally. And, ultimately, these same people are quite likely to tell them that their career will be advanced by writing as well as reading.

There are a great many courses in contemporary clinical education on 'critical appraisal', 'how to read a paper', 'writing for publication', and so on. Most of these courses lack, but would benefit from, an element of language awareness. They tend to concentrate on other issues – how to tell whether a study is well designed, how to make sense of statistics, and in general things other than the actual process of reading or writing. However, academic text – the pages of the *New England Journal of Medicine*, for example – is arcane and incomprehensible to the novice, and this is because the rules of the language game through which scientific content is mediated are opaque.

Partly also, however, the issue of writing for publication pulls together some of the main strands that I have been attempting to tease out. The fact that academic writing is indeed a rule-governed (or at least a rule-guided) activity, as are other aspects of clinical communication, of course, is one of these strands. But beyond that it brings to the fore two debates central to *Language and Clinical Communication*, and present throughout this book – not that I shall be attempting to offer a definitive answer to these questions.

First, to what extent are 'rules' helpful in language? Are there rules which are sufficiently general to be worth the name, yet sufficiently unknown to be worth teaching? 'Put a full stop at the end of a sentence' is a rule, but not a teaching point for most adults contemplating research careers. And secondly, to what extent does obedience to a set of surface rules actually change the way one thinks about things? Does 'attitude' follow 'behaviour'? If one learns rules about the writing of scientific text, does one think more profoundly about the nature of science?

I have prefaced this chapter with part of a brilliant, teasing piece by one of the great scientific writers, Robert Boyle. In this short extract we see him toying with what we might these days refer to as the intrusion of the self into the scientific report. We all know, do we not, that scientific reports are supposed to be facts, facts and more facts – with the writer acting merely as the humble scribe of nature's truths. And we all know – or at least anyone who has ever written for publication knows – that this is not the way it works, that science is written by individuals as venal or virtuous, as altruistic or egotistical, as self-effacing or self-advertising, as one finds in any discipline or none. And, as we see Boyle also looking at the difference between theory and experiment, we see him talking, in a clever and beautifully balanced manner, about how science comes into being.

As with other chapters in this book, I have concentrated in what follows on the teaching side of things, on exercises designed to promote self-awareness, and the ability to talk about things which is at the heart of self-reflection.

Rules and guesses

Language has, say, 'grammar rules.' For example, in English we can say 'I have two brothers' or '. . . a new car' or '. . . a cunning plan', or pretty much anything. On the other hand, we can only say 'I'm having' with reference to a very limited range of things – for instance, 'I'm having a bath', or '. . . lunch' or '. . . a great time.' Now, as with any grammar rule, this doesn't always work – there are regional variations. For example, South Asian English tends to allow wider use of 'I'm having', but by and large the rule is secure enough to teach people as good practice. People are aware of some of these rules ('You go', but 'he goes'), but not others ('big red car', but not 'red big car').

'Grammar' is about the way in which sentences are constructed. However, it is being increasingly appreciated that language also has patterns in units which are bigger than sentences. It's just that these patterns are more difficult to detect, and much less secure than pieces of grammar. As I have said, they are best thought of as tendencies rather than rules.

So, for example, hearing one word or phrase often allows us to predict what will come next. The standard texts exemplify this with phrases which everyone knows – 'kith' is always followed by 'and kin', 'hook, line' is always followed by 'and sinker' – but this is something which pervades languages. For example, in English, a 'defeat' is usually 'heavy', not 'big.' Meat can be 'off', but bread is 'stale', and not the other way round.

Teaching how to write in a genre such as the 'academic article' is therefore concerned with making people aware of the general principle of language as being rule or tendency governed, and of making them more conscious both of what the rules are, and of how to follow them. Again, we do not reinterpret the world from moment to moment. We take short cuts, recognise familiar patterns and make assumptions. In this respect, the good reader knows that text can be predicted.

Indeed, so far as basic reading is concerned, it has long been recognised that the efficient reader does not painstakingly read one word at a time. Reading is, in one of the most famous phrases ever written about it, 'a psycholinguistic guessing game.'[2] We could all complete a sentence like:

> The cat sat on the . . .

We know that the sentence cannot be 'The cat sat on the identify' (because it is not grammatical), we know that it is unlikely to be 'The cat sat on the Tuesday' (because that implies a meaning for the word 'sit' not applied to cats, e.g. 'the court sat on the Tuesday'), we know that it probably isn't 'The cat sat on the zebra' (because our knowledge of the world tells us this seldom happens), and we are likely to guess 'The cat sat on the mat' because our cultural knowledge reminds us that that this is a common display sentence, formerly used for teaching reading to young children and getting them to associate the letter shapes of '-at' with the sound in the words 'cat', 'mat,' etc. And, as I am clearly setting up a display sentence myself, you are moderately likely to guess this way here. Other guesses – unless you were being wilful! – will have been guided by grammar (after 'on the' there must be either a noun or an adjective plus noun) and real-world knowledge (cats tend to sit on chairs, tables, window ledges, and so on).

Understanding special types of reading and writing, such as academic writing, involves applying fundamentally the same principles.

Here is an outline plan of an afternoon's session in 'Teaching Academic Writing'.

Lesson plan

Stage 1   15 minutes

Making guesses

Complete the following sentences:

Give the dog a _____
Ask a stupid _____
How many times do I have to _____
A fool and _____
Yesterday I went to town and_____

This exercise is designed to show a number of things:
- language can be guessed at . . .
- . . . but to variable extents (these sentences are increasingly difficult to complete with certainty)
- as participants will often try to offer amusing examples ('Give the dog a boot up the backside', and so on), the sentences can

be used to demonstrate the way that creativity essentially means successfully extending or breaking conventions.

Can you think of examples of other conventions? What do you say when you see someone in the morning? How do you take your leave from a party? What are you allowed, and not allowed, to discuss with strangers? Politics? People's salaries? The weather?

What conclusions can participants draw?

Stage 2   20 minutes

Shannon's game

Invent a version of a fairy story, and tell the group 'I'm going to give you the first word of a fairy story, and I want you to guess the next word, then the next word, and so on.'

Write the story up on the board as the participants make guesses.

Opening sentence (this example is very roughly based on the opening of *Don Quixote*[3]):

Once – upon – a – time – in – a – land – whose – name – I – do – not – remember – there – lived – long – ago – a – certain – knight

Ask: Were some words easier to guess than others? Why? What conclusions do you draw?

Stage 3   30 minutes

Move structure

Ask the group to think about the Introduction to an academic article – in the *British Medical Journal*, say.

Ask: What do you expect to find in the Introduction? (In groups, report back.)

And what do you expect to find in the Discussion?

Stage 4   90–120 minutes

The proverbs game: an elementary exercise in reading, writing and epistemology

(This exercise is suitable for groups of 3 to 6 participants, or for self-study.)

Write an outline academic article, with a maximum of 800 words, in which you describe an imaginary experiment designed to test one of the following hypotheses:

■ A stitch in time saves nine.

■ The toast always lands butter-side down.

■ Too many cooks spoil the broth.

■ Fine words butter no parsnips.

■ It's an ill wind that blows nobody any good.

Then circulate your paper to other groups and/or present it to them, defending the decisions you made with regard to methodology and choice of language.

Comments on lesson plan

Stage 1 consists of sensitisation exercises only, which are, I hope, self-explanatory.

Stage 2 (Shannon's game) is a standard game (more commonly used to help people with spelling, but it works just as well when used at word level, as here) designed to demonstrate the predictability of text, and to encourage people to guess.

The first four words are very easy – people guess them immediately. And at this stage they will stop. However, a few moments of guesses thrown out from the floor will quickly reveal how limited the options are. In general, guesses will cluster round something like:

in a far-off/strange land

and also something like:

there lived a king/beautiful princess/knight/dragon.

And of course both are likely to come, in one order or the other. The word 'whose' is not usually guessed – it's a slightly rare construction, to have an inanimate noun such as 'land' referred to as 'whose.'

In my experience, this exercise works extremely well with postgraduate groups, who quickly see the serious point behind the game and can extrapolate from it to their own academic writing. (I've been playing Shannon's game for many years with groups at all levels – you get variations that reflect current fashions. 'In a galaxy far, far away' featured heavily at one time, hobbits more recently, and the characters of the Harry Potter books are now beginning to creep in.)

The point is to say that just as words like 'princess' and phrases like 'once upon a time' are the conventions of the fairy story, so there are also conventions in academic writing. These conventions form the bare bones of the paper, and the actual study is the way in which these bones are fleshed out.

The main impetus for work on the research article came from Swales, developed through the 1980s,[1] and considerably extended since then. What I outline below is a modified version of Swales which I have applied elsewhere,[5] and the use of the word 'move', to indicate an identifiable section of text, is taken from him.

Note that because we are dealing here with tendencies, not rules, participants will have no difficulty in finding counter-examples to what is suggested. In fact the important point is to raise awareness, to enable people to look at text in this kind of way, rather than attempting certainty. However, if participants *write* in the way suggested, they will structure their work well. This raises the issue of what sort of status Swales' original work has as 'research.' It has clear *value*, as a structure for teaching, but it is important not to make great claims for the purely *evidential* basis of the patterns that he found. This matters little in language studies, where patterns tend to be poorly defined, because language is like that. (Note the difference here between teaching academic writing and spoken communication. The things which are of sufficient generality to be considered rules are not usually too obvious to be taught.)

Interestingly, the 'Instructions to Authors' pages of many leading journals have now caught up with the research, and what is presented here is, to variable extents, simply an exemplification of what they require, together with a sketch of the psycholinguistic justification behind it. This can of course be drawn to the attention of participants, probably at the end of the session. Note that generalisations about structure are easier to apply to the Introduction and Discussion, where the words on the page are less driven by the nature of the research methodology.

A research paper usually has well-defined sections. Most healthcare professionals can recall that these are – although the labels vary slightly, of course – Introduction, Methods, Results, Discussion (plus Abstract, References, Acknowledgements, and so on). This is known as the 'IMRAD' format, with the 'A' rather feebly standing for 'and.'

What, then, typically goes into an Introduction? If you divide a class of healthcare professionals, at any level, into small groups and ask them, they are likely to come up with the answer you are looking for, which is illustrated in the following example, taken from a *British Medical Journal* paper.[6]

First (Move 1), there's an assertion that something is *important, central, common* or the like. This move can be identified by the appearance of these words or something similar or, as in the example below, by reference to important agencies:

> United Nations' agencies, governmental and non-governmental institutions, professionals and scientists have for many years emphasised the importance of breast feeding for the optimal growth and development of children.

There is then a brief discussion (Move 2) of research, recognisable by the appearance, obviously, of superscript numbers. This paper is rare in having a single such reference at this stage:

> In 1981, the World Health Assembly adopted the International Code of Marketing of Breastmilk Substitutes as a minimum international standard to ensure the proper use of breast milk substitutes.[1]

Then (Move 3) there is an indication of a gap in knowledge, signalled by a word or phrase such as *but, however, little is known, there are few examples*, etc.

> By 1996, all member states had affirmed their support for the adoption of national legislation or other suitable measures to give effect to the principles of the code. In West Africa, few countries have adopted national policies to implement these principles. This is of concern as recent findings suggest that bottle feeding is being encouraged by the increased value placed on 'modern' behaviours and through contact with western health practices, exposure to mass media, and aggressive marketing of breast milk substitutes.[2]

The second reference at this stage is unusual, and the lengthy Move 3 is itself a little unusual. However, we are dealing with tendencies, not rules.

Move 4 makes a statement about the aims of the present study, and is signalled by, for example, a word or phrase such as *This study, We aim*, etc.

> We monitored compliance with the code in Togo, a country without legislation in accordance with the code, and Burkina Faso, which has legislation regulating the marketing of breast milk substitutes.

And what about the Discussion section?

I shall continue to use the same paper, for ease of reference, but have not cited more than the immediately relevant phrases.

The Discussion consists of the following:

■ a restatement (the first move in the Discussion, or Move D1) of the main findings, with a word like *shows, finds, demonstrates*, etc.

> The evidence from this large systematic survey of health facilities, distribution points, health providers, and mothers in Togo and Burkina Faso show that in West Africa . . .

- acknowledgment of weaknesses (Move D2). Interestingly, this is often accompanied by an add-on sentence, introduced by *however*, which restates the paper's claim to value. This particular paper, even more interestingly, has no admission of weaknesses – a clear sign that the purpose of the paper is to drive political change. There is therefore no Move D2
- a recontextualisation in the literature (Move D3) with a phrase like *in accord with, confirms*, etc., and the appearance of superscript numbers again. In this paper, there are six such references to what the situation is in other parts of the world, concluding:

> Using standardised survey methods, we have shown that breast milk manufacturers are also violating the code in Togo and Burkina Faso.

- recommendations for either a change in clinical practice, or an area that requires future research, with an indication of what *should/ought to* happen, or what the authors *suggest* or *recommend*.

In this very political paper, all of the recommendations are for real-world change, there are many of them, and they are unusually forceful:

> This situation requires urgent policy action . . .

> Governments have an obligation to ensure . . .

> Health professionals must support the code.

> Manufacturers have an obligation to comply . . .

> [Manufacturers] should not use healthcare systems to provide mothers with free samples . . .

> Manufacturers must not use distribution points . . .

> [Manufacturers] must stop using the news media to idealise the use of breast milk substitutes.

> Lastly, [manufacturers] must label their products according to the directives of the code.

Once more, groups of health professionals are likely to surprise themselves by how well they can identify, in advance, with a fair bit of reflection, 'the things that a Discussion is likely to contain.'

With regard to the proverbs game (Stage 4), here is a sample answer, for simplicity keeping numerical values at the level of basic arithmetic, ducking the issue of trial type, and retaining only the major IMRAD sections. Therefore I don't go into detail about the sample population, the setting, and so on, although it is possible to do so. (I have published a version of 'Fine words butter no parsnips' elsewhere.[7])

Does a stitch in time save nine? The implications for female polyester-mix clothing of mending or not mending torn garments

Introduction

Many households in the UK suffer from severe financial constraint (ref.). It has been shown that the traditional practice of mending torn or worn garments for reasons of economy is increasingly rare (ref.), and that knowledge of how to make do and mend is deteriorating from generation to generation (ref.). However, no attempt has been made to quantify the extent to which leaving garments unmended undermines their integrity as items of clothing: the view that prompt action results in a ninefold saving is not evidence based, and no time limit is specified for savings to reach this level. This study therefore looked at the effect of prompt stitching on a common garment.

Methods

A total of 1000 letters were distributed to females aged 40–50 years randomised from GP practices in the West Midlands NHS region of the UK. The letter also asked (1) whether the recipient was a UK dress size 12 or 14 (on a good day), and (2) whether they would describe themselves as a 'frequent wearer' of cardigans. The first 200 respondents who matched the inclusion criteria were entered into the study. Inclusion criteria for age and dress size were designed to act as a proxy control for levels of physical activity, which it was hypothesised might impact on levels of wear and tear on the garment.

A total of 200 cardigans made of polyester mix were purchased from a well-known department store, 100 each in UK standard size 12 and size 14. In each case, a small incision was made on the front lower right quadrant, 1/8 inch in length. A total of 50 size 12 cardigans and 50 size 14 cardigans were then designated as intervention cardigans (ICs), and a single stitch was administered. The remaining control cardigans (CCs) were left untreated. Participants were then assigned to an IC or CC, and told to wear it 'as they usually would' for a period of 14 days. The study took place in January, when it was considered that cardigan wearing would reach its annual peak.

The statistical methods used were based on primary school arithmetic.

Results

Two garments (IC = 1, CC = 1) were washed by absent-minded participants, and a further four garments (IC = 3, CC = 1) suffered domestic feline degradation (DFD) during the course of the experiment. Moreover, one garment (CC) was left behind when its owner went on holiday to Dubai, although the participant reported retrospectively that she would have felt the benefit, what with the air-conditioning in the hotel that she hadn't made allowance for, and it getting a bit nippy in the evening. One participant in the CC group had mended her cardigan after 9 days, on the grounds that she couldn't stand it any longer. This potentially age-specific behaviour led us to check her entry profile, and it was discovered that she was in fact 62 years old. All of these cardigans were excluded, leaving 46 IC and 46 CC garments at the end of the experimental period.

The mean length of tear at 14 days was 0.68 inches for the IC group, and 2.2 inches for the CC group. We thought that this was a considerable difference. The additional stitches required to secure the garments such that no tear existed were 188 (mean 4.09) for the CC group, and 732 (mean 15.91) for the IC group. Thus, over a 14-day period, a stitch in time saved 11.82.

Discussion

This study has demonstrated substantial savings of wool over a 14-day period as a result of prompt stitching. This is in accord with findings from folklore (ref.). However, there are a number of limitations to the study. The size of the tear relative to the single stitch administered in the IC group may have impacted on the IC:CC ratio over the study period. That is, with a smaller incision, the mean number of additional stitches may have approached zero, with the ratio approaching infinity. Nor do we know whether the size of the incision increases at a regular rate, allowing extrapolation of these data to longer (or shorter) time periods. There was no difference noted in wear and tear between left- and right-handed participants, although the selection of the front lower right quadrant for the original incision may have favoured left-handed women, who might more frequently use their left arms, and brush against that side of the cardigan more frequently. A larger sample size is needed to resolve this issue, and indeed other demographic variables. Finally, we do not know to what extent the selection of material represents a significant variable.

Nevertheless, we can conclude that there are considerable savings involved in adopting a make-and-mend approach, and recommend it in particular to individuals and groups who are experiencing financial hardship. We believe that there is clearly sufficient evidence now to justify further research into this field.

This is a game that works very well with novice and near-novice researchers.

The ostensible topic for study here is the structure of written academic text in the health sciences, but there is much more to the exercise than this. First, it is impossible to undertake this activity without reflecting on the kind of thing that research involves, and that this experiment (if one was actually to do it) would have to involve. In other words, the general principles are directly in front of the participant, however daft the context. The game sensitises participants intellectually. They find it hard to work at the task without thinking about the nature of science generally.

Secondly, the 800-word example I have given is underwritten (i.e. there is too little detail). However, if there is a time and word limit on the activity, and if people are working in groups to produce a single written version, then the level of detail of my example is already greater than one can normally expect. The advantage of the group is that people will spot methodological problems for each other – the disadvantage is that doing this activity well in fact requires a high level of concentration.

Thirdly, groups or individuals will almost inevitably want to include jokes of some kind, and this helps them to think about what is and is not appropriate academic language. Some of the jokes will involve the use of clearly inappropriate language (my comments about the woman who went to Dubai and the woman who mended her cardigan), some will emphasise the use of appropriate language in a banal or preposterous area (phrases like 'Intervention Cardigans'), and so on.

The game of fraud

The most obvious characteristic of the academic article is perhaps its vocabulary, which is of course highly technical. It is through an understanding of what words are appropriate within the game of 'writing for the health professions' that one can claim membership of the 'discourse community'[8] – that is, the group of people who understand the game, and who are, in the current phrase, 'in the loop.' (For a more detailed discussion of this phrase, see *Language and Clinical Communication*.)

However, if there is a game, then there may be cheats. Not all uses of technical vocabulary are honourable. Some disciplines have a reputation for retreating into windy nonsense. Education, regrettably, is one of these. Perhaps making one's discipline hard to understand is a defence mechanism against enemies (real or imaginary) who might want to claim that one's research was bogus, or at least not 'scientific.'

Making healthcare professionals aware of the possibility of deliberate fraud – or at any rate of presenting their results in a particular light which may not represent the whole truth – is part of an overall drive towards consciousness-raising in the professions. It is this kind of issue which underpins the desire to constrain more and more tightly what one is allowed to say in an academic paper. Thus, for example, journals seem to be moving towards 'Structured Discussions' (with the structure devised and promulgated, however, without reference to any of the research, along the lines first proposed in the applied linguistics literature above). Whether meanings can be constrained in this way is a moot point – it is the nature of scientific enquiry that it ends on a note of speculation, about what *might* be the case rather than what *is* the case – but ultimately the issue is one of accurate reporting of results, and conservative interpretation of them. And the issue is also about avoiding scare stories such as the following[9] (see also Berger and Ioannidis's clever paper[10]):

> Many of us consider science the most reliable, accountable way of explaining how the world works. We trust it. Should we? John Ioannidis, an epidemiologist, recently concluded that most articles published by biomedical journals are flat-out wrong. The sources of error, he found, are numerous: the small size of many studies, for instance, often leads to mistakes, as does the fact that emerging disciplines, which lately abound, may employ standards and methods that are still evolving. Finally, there is bias, which Ioannidis says he believes to be ubiquitous. Bias can take the form of a broadly held but dubious assumption, a partisan position in a longstanding debate (e.g. whether depression is mostly biological or environmental) or (especially slippery) a belief in a hypothesis that can blind a scientist to evidence contradicting it. These factors, Ioannidis argues, weigh especially heavily these days and together make it less than likely that any given published finding is true.

Saddest of all in the annals of obscurantism is the spoof paper[11] submitted by the New York based physicist Alan Sokal to the journal *Social Text*, which created waves around the world – not to mention front page news. Grandly entitled 'Transgressing the boundaries: towards a transformative hermeneutics of quantum gravity', the paper was duly published. By judicious name-dropping of the correct authorities (Derrida, Lacan, Kuhn, Latour), by filling his Bibliography with satisfactory titles ('The irrelevance of reality: Science, ideology and the postmodern universe'), and using a vast number of obscure terms, he buys membership of the discourse community with counterfeit money. Rather neatly and slyly he concludes the paper by acknowledging the help of others, and insisting, as one does, that these others 'are not responsible for any errors or obscurities which may inadvertently remain.'

Here is a brief flavour of the paper, taken from the conclusion (this is one of the easier sections to understand):

> Finally, the content of any science is profoundly constrained by the language within which its discourses are formulated; and mainstream Western physical science has, since Galileo, been formulated in the language of mathematics. But *whose* mathematics? The question is a fundamental one, for, as Aronowitz has observed, 'neither logic nor mathematics escapes the "contamination" of the social.' And as feminist thinkers have repeatedly pointed out, in the present culture this contamination is overwhelmingly capitalist, patriarchal and militaristic: 'mathematics is portrayed as a woman whose nature desires to be the conquered Other.' Thus, a liberatory science cannot be complete without a profound revision of the canon of mathematics. As yet no such emancipatory mathematics exists, and we can only speculate upon its eventual content. We can see hints of it in the multidimensional and nonlinear logic of fuzzy systems theory, but this approach is still heavily marked by its origins in the crisis of late-capitalist production relations.

Sokal's pseudo-argument hinges on his clever and wilful misrepresentation of such matters as the nature of science as a social construct, so that he can happily deny the existence of the real world, and the value of scientific evidence. Yet, as he concludes in his own subsequent discussion of the affair:[12]

> I offered the *Social Text* editors an opportunity to demonstrate their intellectual rigor. Did they meet the test? I don't think so.
>
> I say this not in glee but in sadness. After all, I'm a leftist too (under the Sandinista government I taught mathematics at the National University of Nicaragua). On nearly all practical political issues – including many concerning science and technology – I'm on the same side as the *Social Text* editors. But I'm a leftist (and feminist) *because* of evidence and logic, not in spite of it. Why should the right wing be allowed to monopolize the intellectual high ground?
>
> And why should self-indulgent nonsense – whatever its professed political orientation – be lauded as the height of scholarly achievement?

This is an important moral tale. Sokal's point is ultimately political – a desire to debunk the prevailing relativism of a certain kind of academic discourse, which he associates with 'leftist' politicians, and to reclaim for the left a sense of certainty, a sense that there are things we simply know. (The reader will again recall in this respect the risk that educational constructivism – the province of Dewey and his followers – may be used to foster the crasser forms of 'anything-goes' relativism).

The point I would want to make is different, but I think it has relevance. The secret language of the discourse community – of which 'jargon' is a part – can be used to obscure, to mislead and to get things wrong. Education, as I say, is a case in point, and the literature of education is full of elaborate polysyllabic theory as a result.

References

1 Boyle R. Experiments and considerations touching colours. In: Hunter M, Davis EB, editors. *The Works of Robert Boyle.* London: Pickering and Chatto; 1999 (first published 1664); www.gutenberg.org/etext/14504 (accessed 13 July 2007).

2 Goodman KS. Reading: a psycholinguistic guessing game. *J Read Specialist.* 1967; **6**: 126–35. (Reprinted in Singer H, Ruddeil RB, editors. *Theoretical Models and Processes of Reading.* Newark, DE: International Reading Association; 1976. pp. 497–509.)

3 Cervantes M (Cohen JM, trans.). *The Adventures of Don Quixote.* Harmondsworth: Penguin; 1985 (Part 1 first published in 1605, and Part 2 in 1615).

4 Swales JM. *Genre Analysis: English in academic and research settings.* Cambridge: Cambridge University Press; 1990.

5 Skelton JR. Analysis of the structure of original research papers: an aid to writing original papers for publication. *Br J Gen Pract.* 1994; **44**: 455–9.

6 Aguayo VM, Ross JS, Kanon S *et al.* Monitoring compliance with the International Code of Marketing of Breastmilk Substitutes in West Africa: multisite cross sectional survey in Togo and Burkina Faso. *BMJ.* 2003; **326**: 127–30.

7 Skelton JR. Getting published. In: Carter Y, Thomas C, editors. *Research Methods in Primary Care.* 1997. Oxford: Radcliffe Medical Press; 1997. pp. 167–78.

8 Nystrand M. *What Writers Know: the language, process, and structure of written discourse.* New York: Academic Press; 1982.

9 Dobbs D. Trial and error. *New York Times,* 15 January 2006; www.nytimes.com/2006/01/15/magazine/15wwln_idealab.html?ex=1184472000&en=964f aa5428a5a173&ei=5070 (accessed 13 July 2007).

10 Berger VW, Ioannidis JPA. The decameron of poor research. *BMJ.* 2004; **329**: 1436–40.

11 Sokal AD. Transgressing the boundaries: towards a transformative hermeneutics of quantum gravity. *Social Text.* 1996; **46/47**: 217–52.

12 Sokal AD. A physicist experiments with cultural studies. *Lingua Franca.* 1996; **May/June issue:** 62–4.

CHAPTER 10

The good doctor

Medicine arose out of the primal sympathy of man with man; out of the desire to help those in sorrow, need and sickness.

(William Osler[1])

Context is all

So much for the language games of clinical communication. Now we return to the starting point. The more you know chess, the more you understand what the word 'king' really means in the context of the game. The more you practise as a doctor, the more you understand the word 'diabetes.' The longer you live, the more you understand 'love', or 'ambition', or 'boredom', or the whole gamut of human emotions. These things make sense in context – in the context of a simulation like chess, or the context of our profession, or of our lives. Miss Havisham understands by 'love' something quite different from Darby and Joan, 50 years on and never a cross word. Such are the things that experience and our personalities bring to us.

Context gives meaning. This in the end is the justification for simulation in the professions, and for raising awareness of our understanding of the rules – or at any rate, as appropriate, the conventions and the tendencies – of the games we play. It is also the justification, more locally, for the kind of role-play activity we have discussed in this book, and which is practised so widely and often so well around the world where clinical education is at stake.

The overwhelming importance of context is also, finally, the justification for the involvement of medical humanities in medical education, and both in this book and in *Language and Clinical Communication* I have sought to provide an undercurrent of references to the humanities for this reason.

A good healthcare professional, therefore, is above all someone who understands the context of practice. That is what I think is at the heart of it. The wise professional has an understanding of what they are involved in.

I should like to conclude by taking these ideas a little further.

Describing goodness

I have my own ideas about what good medical practice is. These ideas are closely bound up with my professional predilections, and this clusters round my educational inheritance, which consists essentially of a sense that to strive as a humanist and as an educator is worthwhile. So that, as you see, my personality is also involved, or at least I am inclined to give what I recognise as a personal answer to this question. I also think I understand what *Good Medical Practice*[2] (*see* Box 10.1) means, but only because I work in medical education, because I talk to the people I talk to, I go to the meetings I go to, and can consequently see the working behind the bald statements. To some limited extent (but I'm not a doctor) I know the game.

It isn't that this document – which is required reading for all doctors in the UK, and echoed by similar documents around the world in medicine and beyond – is unclear. And I agree with it all – how could I not? It's simply that, if one reads it on its own, shorn of the context from which it emanates – a complex context full of debates and, sadly, in the UK, of such tragedies as the Shipman affair – it is banal to the point of being unexceptionable, and unexceptionable to the point of being vacuous. At my own Medical School, graduands are required to recite this in place of the Hippocratic Oath, but it has no resonance – these aren't, frankly, words to which someone can commit.

Box 10.1 Good Medical Practice[2]

The duties of a doctor registered with the General Medical Council

Patients must be able to trust doctors with their lives and health. To justify that trust you must show respect for human life and you must:

- make the care of your patient your first concern
- protect and promote the health of patients and the public
- provide a good standard of practice and care
  - keep your professional knowledge and skills up to date
  - recognise and work within the limits of your competence
  - work with colleagues in the ways that best serve patients' interests

- treat patients as individuals and respect their dignity
  - treat patients politely and considerately
  - respect patients' right to confidentiality
- work in partnership with patients
  - listen to patients and respond to their concerns and preferences
  - give patients the information they want or need in a way they can understand
  - respect patients' right to reach decisions with you about their treatment and care
  - support patients in caring for themselves to improve and maintain their health
- be honest and open and act with integrity
  - act without delay if you have good reason to believe that you or a colleague may be putting patients at risk
  - never discriminate unfairly against patients or colleagues
  - never abuse your patients' trust in you or the public's trust in the profession.

You are personally accountable for your professional practice and must always be prepared to justify your decisions and actions.

This is the nature of political statements, indeed perhaps of any kind of effort at formal summary. It has meaning only in context, and means only what those within the loop (the members of the discourse community) understand it to mean. I have no objection to this, and I certainly couldn't improve on the list of duties, but it is what it is – a document that arises and takes meaning from a particular time, place and set of preconceptions. Notice in particular how the articles of the patient-centred faith are sprinkled judiciously throughout – *individuality, politeness, consideration, respect, listening, negotiating, explaining, partnership* . . . these words or their synonyms are all here, as they would be these days, because they are part of our contemporary currency. The concepts will still be here in 50 years, but the ways in which they are expressed may not, perhaps.

The American Medical Association has published similar statements,[3] and specifically invokes the long history of medical ethics. Indeed, all such pronouncements – as the Australian Medical Association, for example, also acknowledges – derive from Hippocrates:

> This Code has grown out of other similar ethical codes stretching back into history, including the Hippocratic Oath.[4]

The invocation of that name, revered over the millennia, instantly reminds us of the constancy of standards, and the mutabilities of their expression. We can no longer subscribe verbatim to every element of the Hippocratic oath, but we feel as if we know what he meant all the same. The General Medical Council statement, the American Medical Association statement, and the similar documents from all over the world – all of these deadly earnest statements, proclamations as significant as any for the profession in our time, are ultimately merely the contemporary shape of an unending desire to understand better how to do things well.

So, then, can we say that context is all? Well, in some ways it is, but the phrase has been a kind of rallying cry over the years for relativism in its various forms. It's the kind of statement which has been used to suggest that there is no such thing as 'absolute knowledge', and in some cases to attempt to undermine the claim of science itself that it can give us an understanding of how things are. In other words, it has been not only an important epistemological issue, but often in more recent eras a rather tiresome one.

My own view, if I can pre-empt what follows, is the traditional one. Some things lend themselves to empirical research, while others do not. The fruits of empirical research give us insight into aspects of the real world, but we can have insight of other kinds into reality from other, non-empirical sources. What matters is that we do not confuse the two. I should add that, in my own areas of expertise, I am often aware that insight from empirical research is a goal not worth pursuing, but that I don't in consequence feel – well – worthless. In particular, with regard to communication, we can isolate bits and pieces which we can test empirically – the presence or absence of skills such as 'asking open questions', and their relationship to higher scores on patient satisfaction questionnaires, and so on. It's just that the empirical bits and pieces amount to much less than the educational whole.

In other words, there isn't always much point in chiselling away at context with all its roughnesses and ambiguities, in the hope that, when all the cutting and paring has been done, some perfect image of the world as it really is will emerge triumphantly from the stone. By this I mean that when it comes to questions such as 'What is a good doctor?', 'What is good clinical communication?' and 'What is good education?', we cannot answer by means of lists, or merely by citing examples, or with certainty, but this does not absolve us from the duty of working vigorously, honestly and intelligently at these very questions. I don't know, ultimately, what a good doctor is – but this doesn't free me from the obligation to ask the question. Or, if you prefer another way of making the point, I regard it as reasonable not to be able to define the concept of a good doctor, but I ought, in my job, to be able to recognise one when I see them.

Good Medical Practice is – and is only, therefore – a list of desirable qualities. Similarly, a few years ago, and rather tongue in cheek, the *British Medical Journal* 'commissioned the finest brains, searched both the "medical literature" and real literature and invited our readers to help us' to answer the questions 'What is a good doctor and how can we make one?'[5] It was, they acknowledged disingenuously, 'a wild goose chase.' Among the contributions from readers – interesting, helpful, well intentioned, good fun, and a wonderful little snapshot of how people articulate such things now, and off the record (that is, away from the *ex cathedra* pronouncements of governments and governing bodies) – were such things as an 'ABC of being a good doctor'.[6] The list – which makes fascinating reading – includes words like 'attentive', 'balanced', 'caring', 'detective', and so on. It includes more than 100 terms, from A to Z as promised, all the way down to 'zestful.' Sadly, there is no 'X', although in today's multicultural world 'xenophile' would do nicely.

Indeed, the correspondence from readers is full of such terms ('learned, honest, kind, humble, enthusiastic . . .'[7]) – commonplace words in one sense, the correspondence which contains them spangled with the small change of virtue. And what do such words mean? Well, that's the crunch. How does one make such words, and such concepts, have real meaning for each of us as individuals? How does one manage to share such meanings beyond oneself? How does one teach them?

Should a doctor act in the patient's interest? It's a question all doctors could answer in their sleep, and how many of us have ever met a doctor who said they didn't? The trouble is that some doctors are morally asleep when they say this. And, for all the caring and sharing terms that are quite properly trotted out when the qualities of the good doctor are discussed, and despite the clear and inescapable references to clinical judgement and competence, there is relatively little about tougher concepts. The virtues that we claim to seek are precisely the caring and sharing virtues which are valued by the age in which we live – a set of compassionate virtues which would once have been described as 'feminine', perhaps. Conceivably one can look at a great deal of the contemporary medical persona (I've drawn attention to the possibility in the teaching of communication[8]) in terms of feminisation, or what might once have been labelled as such. Certainly the virtues thought by previous generations to be 'manly' are seldom mentioned. Toughness, doggedness, courage – the imperturbable, unflappable virtues of a John Buchan hero, not currently in fashion but nonetheless useful – are usually missing. It's a fact which reminds us that lists are transient things, an echo of the times which produce them.

However, with regard to the question of giving simple terms meaning, there are apparently beguilingly simple answers. Or at least, the answer is simple for a humanist. It is indeed to accept that meaning derives from context – that to reduce complex qualities to a list is to end up with less than the sum of the parts. And that to learn oneself and to teach others involves contextual thinking.

For this reason I am doing as the *British Medical Journal* did, and concentrating on what it calls 'real literature', or at any rate, that produced by good writers and profound thinkers. My selection inevitably reflects biases in my own view of professional life, and I have gone out of my way to consider things other than the amorphous desire for empathy in our doctors which is so much in vogue.

Take stoicism, for example, and a kind of dogged willingness not to give up. Doctors make progress slowly, painstakingly and, it might be added, only sometimes.

Here are some brief pictures of doctors, some real and some fictional, and all beautifully written.

Dr Robert Levet was a friend of Dr Samuel Johnson ('Dr' Johnson not as a result of medical training, of course). He was by all accounts an odd man, slightly bizarre perhaps in affect, always short of money, not necessarily as good at his job as Johnson makes him out to be – and he was one of many people whom Johnson took into his household. When he died, Johnson wrote a poem about him – grave, simple and profound, one of the best eulogies in the language. It is informed by Johnson's own stoic turn of mind. The poem is, incidentally, the source of the phrase 'The power of art without the show.' It in fact refers to Levet's qualities as a doctor.

Here is an extract (the word 'officious' as used here means 'fulfilling his duties'):

> Condemn'd to hope's delusive mine,
> As on we toil from day to day,
> By sudden blasts, or slow decline,
> Our social comforts drop away.
>
> Well tried through many a varying year,
> See Levet to the grave descend;
> Officious, innocent, sincere,
> Of ev'ry friendless name the friend.
>
> . . .
>
> In misery's darkest caverns known,
> His useful care was ever nigh,
> Where hopeless anguish pour'd his groan,
> And lonely want retir'd to die.

No summons mock'd by chill delay,
No petty gain disdain'd by pride,
The modest wants of ev'ry day
The toil of ev'ry day supplied.

His virtues walk'd their narrow round,
Nor made a pause, nor left a void;
And sure th' Eternal Master found
The single talent well employ'd.[9]

Dr Levet was not a man of undue learning, as Johnson acknowledges, nor yet of great sophistication, but his steady application to duty – his acceptance of the drudgery that goes with the vocation – is deeply impressive.

Among fictional doctors, Albert Camus' Dr Rieux, who struggles through a plague epidemic as it hits the Algerian city of Oran, demonstrates some of the same qualities with which Johnson imbues Dr Levet, or perhaps more exactly with which he imbues the world through which Dr Levet moves. Dr Rieux is the narrator of Camus' *The Plague*,[10] but – a sign perhaps of his lack of ego – does not make this clear to the reader (the story is told in the third person) until almost the end of the book. One of the triumphs of the novel is, strangely, that Dr Rieux's efforts help only a little. It takes him a long time to persuade the authorities that there is a problem, and his attempts to alleviate the death and suffering which quickly engulf the stricken town seem to make little difference. The world view is bleak, yet one never feels that Rieux has failed. On the contrary, he has heroic stature because he recognises the futility of his efforts, and yet perseveres with them, and with his duty. Early on, when he first appreciates the possibility of plague, he stands at his window, his mind filled with similar horrors in other places:

Athens, a charnel house reeking to heaven and deserted even by the birds; Chinese towns cluttered up with victims silent in their agony; the convicts at Marseille piling up rotten corpses; the building of the Great Wall in Provence to fend off the furious plague wind; . . . nights and days filled always, everywhere, with the eternal cry of human pain.

But eventually:

The doctor pulled himself back from the window, and at once the noises of the town grew louder. The brief, intermittent sibilance of a machine-saw came from a nearby workshop. Rieux pulled himself together. There lay certitude: there, in the daily round. All the rest hung on mere threads and trivial contingencies;

you couldn't waste your time on it. The thing was to do your job as it should be done.

This is what duty is.

The good doctor has always, I suspect, been envisaged as something more than a good clinician, an unerring diagnostician, the surgeon with a finely wielded scalpel – just as the bad doctor has often been envisaged not so much as clinically incompetent, but as a charlatan, a rogue, a man obsessed with cash or social cachet. In this respect it is interesting to note how the backdrop to the debate about professional 'goodness' differs between the USA and other countries. In the USA, the good professional is often seen as under threat not generally, or not merely, from (say) laziness, or a general indifference to the well-being of patients, but specifically is seen as under the threat imposed by 'the market.' This is a contemporary version of the venal rogue who is sprinkled through the pages of literature, although as Rothman[11] points out, with the contemporary 'focus on the threats from managed care' being so 'intense' it is difficult to answer 'the thorny question of whether professionalism is more or less vibrant or effective today than it was.' (It is worth noting that one of Dr Levet's qualities, referred to above, is that money is not his motive – lack of desire for gain is one of his virtues.)

On the other hand, perhaps among our thoughts of medical perfection there has always been a desire for mystery – for a secret, weighty knowledge of drugs, or spells and potions, as the times dictated. Conceivably we imagine an impossible, distant wisdom. Imhotep, maybe – the great Egyptian polymath who is credited among other things with designing the step pyramid at Saqqara, the earliest genius whose name we know, and as Osler states in the lecture quoted above, 'The first figure of a physician to stand out clearly from the mists of antiquity.' (He was, incidentally, like Asclepius, awarded the status of the god of medicine after his death, thus presumably defining an upper limit to medical ambition.)

However, elements of Osler's 'primal sympathy' are also part of our image – or I would argue that they ought to be, provided always that we understand what Osler means. The phrase is in fact Wordsworth's,[12] and Osler goes on to quote the last lines of the relevant stanza in his address:

> What though the radiance which was once so bright
> Be now for ever taken from my sight,
> Though nothing can bring back the hour
> Of splendour in the grass, of glory in the flower;
> We will grieve not, rather find

Strength in what remains behind;
In the primal sympathy
Which having been must ever be;
In the soothing thoughts that spring
Out of human suffering;
In the faith that looks through death,
In years that bring the philosophic mind.

Wordsworth's 'Ode: intimations of immortality' is about growing up, about leaving the easy 'radiance' and 'splendour' of childhood behind, and developing maturity. And a version of professional maturity – here and most famously in his best known piece, 'Aequanimitas' – is Osler's theme, too.[13]

His audience is a group of medical students who are just embarking on their careers. I have removed a number of his classical allusions, since to the modern ear they give an over-ornamented feel to his prose.

> . . . an inscrutable face may prove a fortune. In a true and perfect form, imperturbability is indissolubly associated with wide experience and an intimate knowledge of the varied aspects of disease. With such advantages he is so equipped that no eventuality can disturb the mental equilibrium of the physician; the possibilities are always manifest, and the course of action clear. From its very nature this precious quality is liable to be misinterpreted, and the general accusation of hardness, so often brought against the profession, has here its foundation. Now a certain measure of insensibility is not only an advantage, but a positive necessity in the exercise of a calm judgement, and in carrying out delicate operations. Keen sensibility is doubtless a virtue of high order, when it does not interfere with steadiness of hand or coolness of nerve; but for the practitioner in his working-day world, a callousness which thinks only of the good to be effected, and goes ahead regardless of smaller considerations, is the preferable quality.
>
> Cultivate, then, gentlemen, such a judicious measure of obtuseness as will enable you to meet the exigencies of practice with firmness and courage, without, at the same time, hardening 'the human heart by which we live.' In the second place, there is a mental equivalent to this bodily endowment, which is as important in our pilgrimage as imperturbability. Let me recall to your minds an incident related of that best of men and wisest of rulers, Antoninus Pius, who, as he lay dying . . . summed up the philosophy of life in the watchword, *Aequanimitas*. As for him . . . so for you . . . a calm equanimity is the desirable attitude. How difficult to attain, yet how necessary, in success as in failure! Natural temperament has much to do with its development, but a clear

knowledge of our relation to our fellow-creatures and to the work of life is also indispensable.

This is an essay which can cause disquiet. People react badly, if they don't read carefully, to the idea that clinicians ought to be 'inscrutable', that they ought to have a capacity for demonstrating 'insensibility', 'obtuseness', 'imperturbability' – although the meaning of these words has changed somewhat over the last century. They see in these words, in the very terms which Osler uses, a clinician guilty of the 'general accusation of hardness' which he recognises as an occupational hazard. However, it seems to me that professional wisdom – what these days we would call a proper professional attitude – is what is at stake.

The majority of fictional doctors are negatively portrayed. Of those who are not, Charles Dickens' brief sketch of the generically described individual known only as 'Physician', who appears from time to time moving in the world of illusion and deception which is *Little Dorrit*,[14] strikes the perfect note. He is not, I think, the kind of doctor who has chosen to lose himself beneath a weight of ego, but neither is he all gushing empathy:

> Few ways of life were hidden from Physician, and he was oftener in its darkest places than even Bishop. There were brilliant ladies about London who perfectly doted on him, my dear, as the most charming creature and the most delightful person, who would have been shocked to find themselves so close to him if they could have known on what sights those thoughtful eyes of his had rested within an hour or two, and near to whose beds, and under what roofs, his composed figure had stood. But Physician was a composed man, who performed neither on his own trumpet, nor on the trumpets of other people. Many wonderful things did he see and hear, and much irreconcilable moral contradiction did he pass his life among; yet his equality of compassion was no more disturbed than the Divine Master's of all healing was. He went, like the rain, among the just and unjust, doing all the good he could, and neither proclaiming it in the synagogues nor at the corner of streets.
>
> As no man of large experience of humanity, however quietly carried it may be, can fail to be invested with an interest peculiar to the possession of such knowledge, Physician was an attractive man. Even the daintier gentlemen and ladies who had no idea of his secret, and who would have been startled out of more wits than they had, by the monstrous impropriety of his proposing to them 'Come and see what I see!', confessed his attraction. Where he was, something real was. And half a grain of reality, like the smallest portion of some other scarce natural productions, will flavour an enormous quantity of diluent.

I have focused part of this brief discussion on Osler because he himself has often been held up as the exemplar for the good doctor – and perhaps this is appropriate. At any rate, the point is that our paragon is somebody, not nobody – a person, not a list of attributes – by which I mean that he or she will have clinical expertise allied to a seriousness and sincerity of purpose, a maturity and depth of character. In short, the good doctor has a grown-up personality.

This is the grand design. These days, to this kind of elemental picture, one would be likely to add phrases from the litany of contemporary educational virtues – patient-centredness, self-reflection, empathy, and the like – and, of course, good communication skills. Here is one carefully crafted definition of 'professionalism', from Epstein and Hundert,[15] a formidably thorough review of the definition and assessment of professional competence. We may perhaps take 'professional' in this context to be another way of saying 'good.'

> . . . we propose that professional competence is *the habitual and judicious use of communication, knowledge, technical skills, clinical reasoning, emotions, values and reflection in daily practice for the benefit of the individual and community being served*. Competence builds on a foundation of basic clinical skills, scientific knowledge and moral development. It includes a cognitive function – acquiring and using knowledge to solve real-life problems; an integrative function – using biomedical and psychosocial data in clinical reasoning; a relational function – communicating effectively with patients and colleagues; and an affective/moral function – the willingness, patience and emotional awareness to use these skills judiciously and humanely. Competence depends on habits of mind, including attentiveness, critical curiosity, self-awareness and presence. Professional competence is developmental, impermanent and context-dependent.

Of the relevant 'dimensions' into which professionalism is subdivided, there are two which interest us, namely the 'Relationship' dimension and the 'Affective/ Moral' dimension, which break down as follows:
- Relationship:
  - communication skills
  - handling conflict
  - teamwork
  - teaching others (e.g. patients, students and colleagues).
- Affective/moral:
  - tolerance of ambiguity and anxiety
  - emotional intelligence
  - respect for patients

▪ responsiveness to patients and society
▪ caring.

These terms are unexceptionable, but a lot of them show signs of being a vocabulary impoverished by academic handling, virtues hardened into constructs, an ideal splintered into an approximation of its component parts. This is why I have tried to set my arguments against a straightforwardly humanistic backdrop.

Here, by way of alternative, is the voice of an individual doctor talking about a patient whom he admires. It brings the construct to life, gives context to the concept, and stresses qualities not quantities:

> There's magic moments in the in the career of a doctor. Meeting her was one of them y'know it's a very privileged situation to be there, to be able to [go] into that family situation to be to know all the details and to be involved y'know and to see the courage and it's it has to be courage really phenomenal courage to see that in action y'know . . . and I'm interested to see her wit and her humour her character and that y'know. So I think that that's [a] real privilege for me to be in in there and I think part of the secret of surviving as a family doctor I think is to . . . well it's to treasure those moments y'know I think it's a wealth of treasure y'know unfortunately . . . there there is a tendency in our job to quantify in terms of policy and expense when in actual fact it's not like that y'know it's a way of life.

(Data courtesy of Irish College of General Practice, and Dr M O'Riordan)

My point is this. The 'dimensions' are perhaps as good as it gets when it comes to formulating an abstract definition of the good doctor. However, on their own they mean little. They must echo in the heart and spirit of the doctor who knows the game. And when it comes to teaching them, the point is that what cannot be easily defined, easily researched or easily analysed, can be demonstrated.

References

1 Osler W. *The Evolution of Modern Medicine. A series of lectures delivered at Yale University on the Silliman Foundation in April 1913*. New Haven, CT: Yale University Press; 1921. pp. 196–7; www.encyclopediaindex.com/b/teomm10. htm (accessed 13 July 2007).

2 General Medical Council. *Good Medical Practice*. London: General Medical Council; 2006; http://gmcuk.org/guidance/good_medical_practice/index.asp (accessed 13 July 2007).

3 American Medical Association; www.ama-assn.org/ama/pub/category/8291. html (accessed 21 February 2007).

4 Australian Medical Association; www.ama.com.au/web.nsf/tag/amacodeofethics (accessed 21 February 2007).

5 The BMJ's wild goose chase. *BMJ*. 2002; **325**: i.

6 Parmar MS. ABC of being a good doctor. *BMJ*. 2002; **325**: 711–12.

7 Sotelo J. Good doctors abound. *BMJ*. 2002; **325**: 712.

8 Skelton JR, Hobbs FDR. Girl talk: co-operative language and physician gender in the primary care consultation. *BMJ*. 1999; **318**: 576–9.

9 Johnson S (Greene D, editor). *The Major Works*. Oxford: Oxford University Press; 2000 (written 1783). p. 35.

10 Camus A (Gilbert S, trans.). *The Plague*. Harmondsworth: Penguin; 1960 (first published 1947). pp. 36–7.

11 Rothman DJ. Medical professionalism – focusing on the real issues. *NEJM*. 2000; **342**: 1284–6.

12 Wordsworth W. Ode: intimations of immortality. In: Gill S, editor. *Wordsworth: the major works*. Oxford: Oxford University Press; 2000. pp. 297–302. (First published as: Ode (There was a time), in 1807.)

13 Osler W. *Aequanimitas*. In: Osler W. *Aequanimitas with Other Addresses to Medical Students, Nurses and Practitioners of Medicine*. 3rd ed. New York: McGraw Hill; 1932. (Valedictory address, University of Pennsylvania, 1 May 1889.)

14 Dickens C. *Little Dorrit*. Harmondsworth: Penguin Classics; 2003 (first published 1857).

15 Epstein RM, Hundert M. Defining and assessing professional competence. *JAMA*. 2002; **287**: 226–35.

Appendix

A note on the database

For examples I have drawn from the Birmingham Database of General Practice Consultations built up between 1993 and 1995, and reported, for example, in Skelton and Hobbs.[1] In total there are 373 consultations, with 40 doctors. The database is now too elderly, I think, to be used without reservation as evidence of contemporary practice, and I have tried to draw on it only in order to illustrate points which are relatively resistant to the vagaries of time.

Transcription conventions

Most transcription conventions derive ultimately from those developed by Gail Jefferson, and applied by the sociolinguists of the 1960s. Jefferson's conventions are conveniently available in Atkinson and Heritage.[2] The conventions used here are in part adapted from these, in a very much simplified form.

It goes without saying that any transcription is imperfect, and loses a great deal of what has happened.

1 All pronunciations are regularised to standard UK English, except for a few marginal cases. *Yeah*, *gonna*, *dunno*, *nope* are all recognised. Brief interjections are regularised to *hmm*, *erm* and *uhm*.

2 Only names in the public domain appear. Otherwise, <*Fir*> appears for a first name, and <*Fam*> for a family name. Where more than one such name occurs, they are numbered <*Fir1*>, etc.

3 Where there is a clearly wrong pronunciation (e.g. of a drug name), the mistaken pronunciation is rendered thus: {*stepascope*} (for 'stethoscope'). Only letters of the Roman alphabet are used to capture pronunciations.

Where a speaker embarks on a word and abandons it, this appears in the text as, for example, '*I und[erstand] I know what you mean, doctor.*' If the abandoned word cannot be identified with certainty, it appears as, for example, '*I [zzz] I know what you mean, doctor.*'

4 Silences of 1 second or more are rendered as, for example, *<silence12>*, indicating a silence of 12 seconds. Silences of less than 1 second are ignored.

5 Certain non-language activities are recognised, for example *<laugh>*, *<cry>*, *<write>*, where the activity is of duration more than 1 second. As above, the duration is written in numerals following the descriptive term. Physical examinations are rendered as *<PhysS>* at the beginning, *<PhysF>* at the end. Categories such as *<write>* are only included if the transcriber (who has access to tape only) is certain of the activity.

6 Interruptions, or any instance of two people's speech overlapping, are recognised by an oblique at the end of the word during which the overlap begins. In the interests of readability, a series of short interjections by a second speaker, such as repeated '*hmm*'s, are placed together at the end of the first speaker's turn, thus:

> *Patient:* So I've been feeling/a bit down doctor/, really fed up.
>
> *Doctor:* /Hmm/hmm. I'm sorry to hear it.

References

1 Skelton JR, Hobbs FDR. Concordancing: use of language-based research in medical communication. *Lancet.* 1999; **353**: 108–11.

2 Atkinson J, Heritage J, editors. *Structures of Social Interaction: studies in conversation analysis.* London: Collins; 1987.

Index